Fluids and Electrolytes

An Easy and Intuitive Way to Understand and Memorize Fluids, Electrolytes, and Acidic-Base Balance.

By

Nathan Orwell

Discover the Entire Collection!

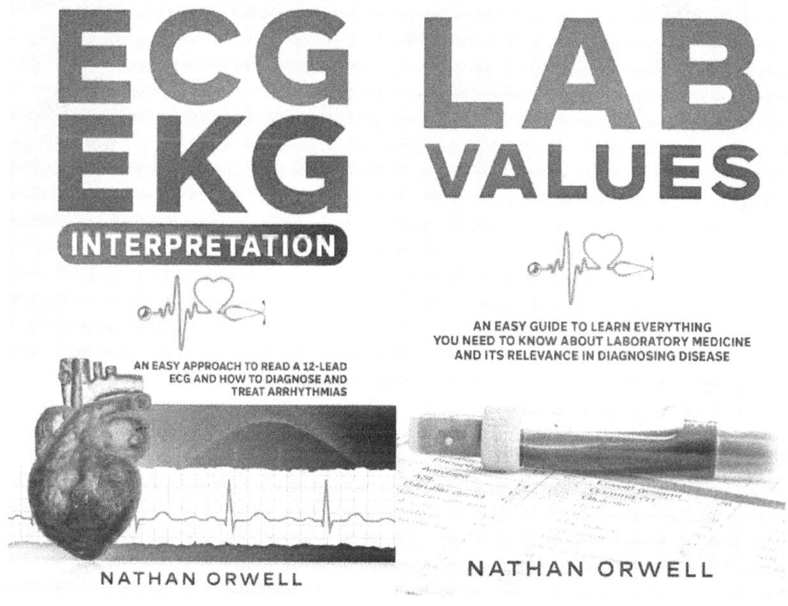

Table of Contents

TABLE OF CONTENTS 6

CHAPTER 1 8

1.0 BODY FLUIDS OR BIOFLUIDS 8

CHAPTER 2 27

2.0 BODY FLUIDS AND COMPARTMENTS 27

CHAPTER 3 78

3.0 SERUM POTASSIUM 78

CHAPTER 4 91

4.0 SERUM PHOSPHATE 91

CHAPTER 5 103

5.0 SERUM SODIUM 103

CHAPTER 6 118

6.0 SERUM MAGNESIUM 118

CHAPTER 7 137

7.0 SERUM CALCIUM 137

CHAPTER 8 149

8.0 SERUM CHLORIDE 149

CHAPTER 9 164

9.0 ARTERIAL BLOOD GASES 164

CHAPTER 10 175

10.0 CAUSES OF ACID-BASE DISTURBANCES 175

Chapter 1

1.0 Body Fluids or Biofluids

Biofluids or body fluids are the main fluid components in the body that contribute to all the regulatory and metabolic activities in the body. As far as all humans are living, the body fluids do not stop circulating. The circulation, composition, and style of activities vary. Moreover, this is the motive why it is necessary to study the mode of circulation and "what body fluids imply in reality."

In an adult human, the amount of biofluids should be at the average level of 60% of the total body weight. The amount of water level in males and females differs. While the male measures are between 60% - 67%, the female one is slightly below this range. Another case is the study of biofluids via the measures of **body fat.** Body fat measure is proportional to body fluids in an inverse manner. Furthermore, this is crucial to measures the number of biofluids and the composition of the body fluids.

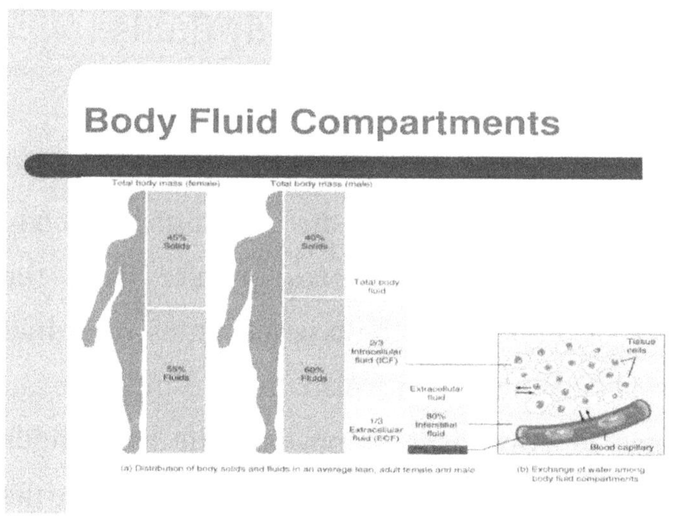

Biofluids are grouped into two categories; *"extracellular and intracellular fluids."* The grouping is analyzed based on the position of the fluids, the composition, and the presence/absence of some particles or determinants. Based on composition, the extracellular fluids are grouped into *interstitial fluids and intravascular fluids.*

- **Extracellular fluid**
    - *Intervascular fluid*
    - *Intravascular fluid*
    - *Lymphatic fluid*
    - *Transcellular fluid*

- **Intracellular fluid**

1.1 Health Significance of Body fluids

Body fluids are significant to the medical world. One of the health practice measures is the implications of body fluids in monitoring sicknesses' nature and the importance of pinpointing the type of illness regarding serum tests, among others. Also, body fluids are an indication of opportunistic pathogens. The body fluids give way to vectors, and these pathogens can influence the body without much restriction due to the presence and wide distribution of the pathogens.

Therefore, it is mandatory to know the level of these fluids, their nature, and the composition mode in time intervals. Thus, medical measures like blood-borne and sexually transmitted diseases are infectious illnesses that are confined and monitored via the observation of body fluids. Also, the act of practicing safe sex and precautions, especially in regards to body fluids", is directly related to the practice of avoiding the exchange of body fluids between two individuals (either the same sex or opposite sex).

Health methods of extracting body fluids:

- *Thoracentesis*
- *Lumbar puncture*
- *Venous blood sampling*
- *Arterial blood sampling*
- *Paracentesis*
- *Amniocentesis*

1.2 Basic Concepts of Body fluids

Body fluids – Solutions, Colloids, Osmolality, Electrochemical terms, and Suspensions

This section gives the background knowledge of biofluids. The study and understanding of body fluids require the necessary interpretation and meaning of some terminologies surrounding "solutions, colloids, and suspensions." The three factors contribute to either balanced or unbalanced body fluids in a human. And this further determines the interpretation and type of solutions. All in all, it contributes to the understanding of body chemistry.

1. Solution

The solution is the combination of solutes and solvents. In the body, the amount of solution is known via the interaction of solutes and solvents. The solute-in-solvent dissolution (in the body) determines if the combination is dissolved or suspended solutions. The principal solvent in the body is water, it is widely distributed, and contains various solutes in different parts of the body. Water has direct implications on the behavior of dissolved materials because it is a polar solvent itself. Meaning, water may not be the dissolving vehicle for non-polar solutes. Thus, other solvents in the body are purely non-solvent.

2. Suspension

The suspension is the terminology of a solute that floats in a solvent. In this sense, a solute does not dissolve in the solution. It instead flows and moves in the direction of the solvents. For example, red blood cells do not dissolve in the plasma. It floats and moves in the direction of the plasma.

The state of motion and action shows if the suspended particles settle or keep moving.

3. Colloids

Colloids are water-loving substances. They attract water and become sticky or gel-like. For example, the protoplasm inside the cells is a direct image of colloids. On average, the level of water in such cells or a colloid in the body should be monitored, especially in a patient that has related issues with body fluids. Often, the level of water should not rise to the story of a hypotonic environment.

Body fluids — Basic Concepts

1. Concentration of Solutions

The concentration of a solution is the number of dissolved solutes in a solvent. Although the solvent has significant importance, the measures are basically based on the number of solutes keeping the solvent constant. The act of removing solvent/adding solutes increases the concentration and vice versa.

So, it is mandatory to monitor the situation whereby a patient may contribute to an increase/decrease in fluid concentration at a particular point in time. Some of the fluid concentrations are urine concentration, blood concentration, sugar concentration, among others.

The concentration is affected by temperature and pressure. Thus, they determine the solubility of a fluid.

- **Saturated solutions** happen when the maximum amount of a solute has dissolved in a solvent. Meaning, if the additional solute is added to the solvent, it will not dissolve.

- **Supersaturated solutions** occur when the condition is the same, and the solvent has more solute than the saturated solutions.

2. Osmotic Pressure of Solutions

Osmotic pressure, or oncotic pressure, is the force that moves solvents across a semipermeable membrane. The number of solvents and solutes should equal on both sides of the membranes. A semipermeable membrane allows solvents to pass through the membrane and mostly restricts the membrane from allowing solutes to pass. On division, the semipermeable membrane allows the solvent to pass from one side to the other. The usual means imply that the number of molecules passing through one side should equal the other ends. *The change in this state results in an increase in the osmotic pressure.*

When there is a change in the amount of solvents or solute in a solution, the osmotic pressure allows the solvents to pass through the membrane into the solution until the solution becomes an equilibrium across all the membranes. Balance exists when the concentrations in both compartments are equal.

3. Electrochemical representation

Based on electrochemical representation, there are 3 essential kinds of physiologic arrangements. Contingent upon the solute, arrangements are polar, non-polar, and ionic (electrovalent).

In nonpolar covalent arrangements, atoms of solute do not convey electrical charges and remain compact. These arrangements are alluded to as **non-electrolytes**. Non-electrolytes are not pulled in to either the positive or the negative post of an anode (subsequently the name nonpolar). Each of the three sorts of arrangements exists together in the body. These arrangements additionally fill in as the media in which colloids and suspensions are dispensed.

Type of Solution	Description	Typical Examples
Polar	The solution is formed from the ionization of solute in water or other solvents with an end result of ions (cations and anions). Ionized water is a good conductor of electricity, and other solvents may conduct electricity depending on the mode of ionization—strong or weak.	CH_3COOH, HCL
Non-Polar	The solution does not polarize; that is, it is electrically neutral–the number of cations and anions is equal. And it does not conduct electricity.	$C_6H_{12}O_6$

Ionic	The ionic solution is formed from the ionization of solutes in water. The difference from POLAR is the characteristics of the solute—which is usually in crystalline form. Also, it produces high electrolytes and conducts electricity.	0.9% of NaCl

On ionic and polar covalent arrangements, a portion of the solute ionizes into isolated particles — ions. A medium in which this separation happens is called an electrolyte arrangement. In the event that an anode is put in such, positive particles move to the terminal's negative post. These particles are called cations. Negative particles move to the positive side of the anode; they are called anions.

Gases, for example, O_2 and CO_2, are nonpolar atoms (alongside N_2) and do not break down very well in water, which is a polar dissolvable.

4. Rule of Thumb

The arrangement and interactions of hypertonic, hypotonic, and isotonic solutions affect the system. Isotonic is the interaction of osmotic pressure that is equal in measure to the average intercellular pressure in the body. In order to achieve this, both the solution and the environment have to be on the same pressure measures level. An example is the equivalent of a saline solution with 0.9% concentration.

Hypotonic solutions occur when the osmotic pressure concentration is lower than the intracellular pressure in the body. Hypertonic solutions are when the osmotic pressure is higher than the intracellular pressure.

The introduction of isotonic solutions into the body system does not affect fluid concentration. The same is the reason most solutions are prepared in an isotonic state. Hypertonic solutions are not always introduced into the body. The solution takes water out of the cells and increasing the concentration of solutes in the cells. Hypotonic solutions permit water absorption; water is absorbed from the solution into the cells.

5. Tonicity

Tonicity depicts how much a solution exerts osmotic pressure. Normal body cell liquid has tonicity equivalent to a 0.9% arrangement of sodium chloride (NaCl, here and there alluded to as physiologic saline).

Arrangements with comparative tonicity are called isotonic. Arrangements with the greater constitution are hypertonic, while with less constitution are hypotonic. Most cells live in a hypotonic climate in which the grouping of water (solute) is lower inside the cell than in the environmental factors.

Water streams into the cell until the layer limits further extension. Pressure increases inside the cell to balance the osmotic pressing factor. This pressure is called turgor. It keeps excess water from entering the cell layers.

The harmony it creates permits the cell to keep an inclination across the cell film. Some cells have particular penetrability, allowing entry of water as well as of explicit solutes. Through these components, supplements and physiologic arrangements are dispersed all through the body.

6. Osmolality

Osmolality is described as the proportion of solute that is dissolvable in a solvent. In physiology, the solvent is water. 5.7 Osmotic pressing factor relies upon the number of particles in the arrangement, yet not on their charge or personality.

A 2% arrangement has double the osmotic pressing factor of a 1% arrangement under comparable pressing factors. For a given measure of solute, the osmotic pressing factor is contrarily corresponding to the solvent volume. Most cell dividers are semipermeable layers.
Through osmotic pressure, water is disseminated all through the body inside certain physiologic reaches.

1.3 Quantitative analysis of Solute Activity and Content

The amount of solute is easily quantified before the reaction with a solvent, or before dissolution. In common terms, the weight is measured using physical measuring media by *actual weight measurements.*

However, the amount of the reaction or chemical combining power is not easily deduced by physical means.

Chemical combining power is vital in medicine, and the term is used to measure the equivalent weight of solutes in a solution. Based on differences in solution, the equivalent weight of physiologic substances has the same amounts of substances with equal chemical combining power. *For instance, the reaction between two chemicals* ***A & B,*** *implies that exactly one equivalent weight of B reacted with one equivalent weight of A.* The chemical combining the power of solution differs, and the ratio and analysis of equal wcights are used to calculate the chemical combining the power of various substances.

The values of equivalent weight are analyzed on milligram equivalent weight measures **(mEq) and gram equivalent weight (gEq).**

- **Milligram Equivalent Weights (mEq)**

Based on measure, the equivalent amount of gEq to mEq is 0.001gEq = 1mEq. The amount of these measures in the body are relatively small, and most values are expressed in mEq. For example, the amount of serum potassium is 3.5 mEq/L - 5.0 mEq/L. This expression is easy to understand than the expression in grams of 0.0035 gEq/L - 0.005 gEq/L.

- **Gram Equivalent Weight Values (gEq)**

The value of gEq is calculated using the valence of certain electrons that are involved in the process. For example, the valence of an electron can be (+) or (-), and this is the charge on the electrons in their ionic state.

So, gEq is calculated by equating the gram of electrons with the valence.

gEq = Gram molecular weight ÷ Valence

1.4 Solute Content by Weight

Substances in body fluids are minimal. And thus, they are expressed in milligrams. The measures are used to assess the ratio of substances weight and the dissolving solvents. For example, in medicine, the actual weight of importance is measured in milligrams percent or milligrams per deciliter of fluid or milligrams of 100ml of body fluid.

$mEq/L = mEq/L \times Equivalent\ weight/10$

$mEq/L = mg/dl \times 10 Equivalent\ weight$

- *For example,*

  To convert a serum K^+ value of 325 mg/dl to mEq/L;

  $mEq/L = (mg/dl \times 10)/\ Equivalent\ weight$

  $= (325 \times 10)/\ 39$

  $= 83.333\ mEq/L$

Solute content by weight is applicable in medical practices when a medical test shows a deficiency in the number of electrolytes in the body. Then, the use of **Lactated Ringer's solution** is applied to resolved the issue and used mainly for the replacement of the low electrolytes. And this is majorly expressed in mEq/L.

The value of Lactated Ringer's Solution:

Constituting substance	mg/dl	mEq/L
KCl	30 of K	4
$NaC_3H_5O_3$	30 of $C_3H_5O_3$	28
NaCl	600 of Na	130
	310 of Cl	109
CaCl	20 of Ca	27

Other measures are used to evaluate the solute content, especially when there is a need to check the dilution of solutions and solute content.

In the medical series, the number of solute values in the solution can be evaluated as:

- **Normal solution**

Standard solution or normality is the solution that has exactly 1 gram of solutes in 1 liter of the final solution.

- **Weight-per-volume solution**

The weight-per-volume solution is sometimes regarded as a percent solution. The measure is significantly applicable to the weight of solute to the volume of the solution. *Solutes are expressed in grams of 100ml of solution.*
The dissolution of glucose into the water means that a specific weight of glucose is dissolved in 100ml of water. In another sense, liquid dissolved in a liquid is considered as volumes of solute in volumes of solution.

- **Ratio solution**

Solutes and solvents are considered in this sense. The equation or evaluation of the two values in the ratio is called ratio solution. 1g of solutes in 100ml of solvents is called (1: 100) ratio. Ratio solution is majorly used in the preparation of drugs and the evaluation of drug purity.

- **Molal and Molar solution**

Molal solution is expressed as 1 mmol/g of solvent. By definition, the molal solution is the amount of 1 mole of solute dissolved in 1 kilogram of solvent.

The molar solution is different as 1 mole of solute is dissolved in 1 liter of solution. Molar solutions are often prepared instead of a molal solution as the amount of solution is not often beyond the standard and required values of 1 liter of solutions.

- **Percent solution**

Percent solution is a measure of solute's weight and solvent's weight. For example, the weight of solute per solution is called a percent solution. *Saline is 0.9% of the total solution weight of 1000g.*

Chapter 2

2.0 Body Fluids and Compartments

Body Fluids and compartments show the importance of water in our body. How does the water affect the body system? The answer is analyzed in both the intracellular and extracellular sections. The balance of each of the compartments is necessary to understand the importance of water in the body.

Analysis of the intracellular fluid composition with that of the extracellular fluid is outlined in the section. Furthermore, it extends to the explanation of the protein channels in the movement of solutes. The movement of water from the extracellular to the intracellular and vice versa explain edema's causes and symptoms in this chapter.

All the action that is life-based occurs in the aqueous solutions in the body. The solution contains many solutes that are dissolved in the solvent.

The solutes are more than one, and each requires some specific mode of operations — chemical reactions. These solutes are found in many parts of the body, and some are carbohydrates, lipids, proteins, salt, minerals, among others.

Water balances or movement of water across the body happens via the action of transports like osmosis—where water moved across semipermeable membrane following the pattern of the osmotic gradient. Thus, water moves from a low concentration of solutes to a high concentration of solutes. And this ensures the appropriate balance of solutes across the body tissues.

2.1 Water in the body

The body content decreases with age. The infants have approximately 75% water content in their bodies and reduce up to 45% in an old age human. The decrease in water content occurs due to age, development, and changes to the body's organs. Most of the water content is stored in the organs of the body—like, kidneys, muscles, bone, have various water levels in the body. The kidneys and brain have about 80% - 85% of water which is the body's highest water content.

The overall water content in humans varies due to certain conditions like obesity. Obesity reduces the level of water in the body and replaced water with fats. The distribution of water through the body may be affected too, and this can cause imbalances in the quantity of water in the body. For example, all the tissues have different modes and shapes for absorbing surfaces which diseases can influence. Once the tissue is infected, it misbehaves; and, thus, decreasing inefficiency.

2.2 Body Fluid Composition

Fluid composition varies across the membrane. The importance of these fluids occurs regarding the blood. The interaction between fluids in the body and blood determines the composition of the fluid. Meaning, fluid varies across tissues in the body. While some have a high concentration of certain values, others may lack the same values. Thus, compartmentalization contributes to establishing fluid composition in the body because these compartments' walls do not allow easy exchange of fluids across each membrane, thereby maintaining standard or unique composition. Some are listed:

Difference

ECF	ICF
• Most abundant cation - Na+, – muscle contraction – Impulse transmission – fluid and electrolyte balance • Most abundant anion - Cl- – Regulates osmotic pressure – Forms HCl in gastric acid	• Most abundant cation - K^+ – Resting membrane potential – Action potentials – Maintains intracellular volume – Regulation of pH • Anion are proteins and phosphates (HPO_4^{2-})

•Na+ /K+ pumps play major role in keeping K+ high inside cells and Na+ high outside cell

1. Extracellular fluid composition

The significant elements in the extracellular fluid are potassium, sodium, calcium, chlorine, and hydrogen carbonate. Although they exist in ionic forms with varying measures as listed below.

Extracellular fluid measures:

Sodium (Na^+)	135 - 145 mEq/L
Calcium (Ca_2^+)	8.4 - 10.5 mEq/L
Potassium (K^+)	3.5 - 5.5 mEq/L
HCO_3^-	22 - 26 mM
Cl^-	27 mEq/kg

Other substances are dissolved in the extracellular fluids, majorly in the fluid called the **plasma**. Plasma has about 93% of water. It has many elements like hormones, carbon dioxide, clotting factors, glucose, fibrinogens, globulins, and the likes. All these substances partake in various chemical processes in the body and change the immune system function, exchange & assimilation of drugs, and transportation.

In essential terms, the extracellular fluid has an exact composition and level of absorption/release. Any deviation can cause complications and significant health conditions.

2. Intracellular Fluid Composition

Intracellular fluid is not much different from extracellular fluid. The only difference is the composition. While some substances are high/low in the extracellular fluid, the reverse occurs in the intracellular fluid. This is a significant difference that must be maintained and put into check-in all diversification. The intracellular fluid contains dissolved ions, molecules (which can be large or small), water-soluble substances, and water as the primary solvent.

Major enzymes contribute to the change in the intracellular fluid, and thus the action in the intracellular fluid is considered complex compare to the extracellular fluid. Normal reactions require one or more enzyme reactions at different stages of the chemical reaction. The shortage of these enzymes can cause complications.

Intracellular layers are different as some channels are required to transport substances out of the cell. Often, some are trigger-bond. Without these triggers, the cell may not transport substances or perform regular activities. Transport pumps exist in active and passive transport, which are specialized modes of transportation in the intracellular cells.

The dissolved substances level in the intracellular fluid is higher than the extracellular fluid. Thus, major chemical activities and medical complications are linked to the intracellular cell than other parts of the cells.

The cytosol has a high level of proteins, waste products, carbohydrates, and lipids than the extracellular fluid.

In contrast, the extracellular fluid has a high level of potassium ions which instigates the active transport of substances in the cell, often against substances' concentration gradient.

Also, the sodium ion is high in the intracellular fluid; it performs actions similar to the potassium ions (that is, active transport).

The intracellular pH level must be constant also. This is because some enzymes may be inactive in acidic or basic solutions. Thus the pH is relatively neutral with a pH of 7.4. The cytosol contains about 70% water content, with a neutral pH level.

3. Transcellular Fluid Composition

Major electrolytes in the transcellular fluid include bicarbonates ions, chloride ions, and sodium ions. This composition varies across the location of each transcellular fluid. For example, cerebrospinal fluid lacks a particular protein present in other fluids (at least some other fluids). Moreover, a typical instance is the case of albumin. The passage that encompasses the cerebrospinal fluid is too small for the selection of albumin. And Ocular fluid in the eye contains high values of antibiotics—proteins contrarily to cerebrospinal fluid.

2.3 Body Fluids Compartments

Fluid compartments are the various places that each fluid is located in the body. The significance of compartmentalization is to distinguish the fluid necessary for medical use and its composition. Fluids in each compartment do not have the same or similar composition. If not for other reasons, the position of fluids relative to the cells' cellular membrane differentiates the body's fluids.

1. Extracellular Fluid Compartment

The extracellular fluid, by definition, is the fluid that is located out of the cell. There are many cells in the body, and each of these cells has cell membranes. Any fluid located outside these membranes is the extracellular fluid. In medical terms, extracellular fluids include *blood plasma and interstitial fluid*—these are the two main types of extracellular fluid.

The approximate measure of extracellular fluid is about 15L— the plasma takes only 3L, while interstitial fluid has about 12L of the total volume.

The pH of extracellular fluids in humans must be maintained at 7.4, and it is buffer. For example, the glucose concentration of cells is regulated by water-balance to be approximately 5 mm, which is a significant measure to act in the body. Another type of extracellular fluid is the *transcellular fluid* which is about 2.5% of the extracellular fluids.

- **Transcellular fluid**

The transcellular fluid includes the plasma and interstitial fluids. It is the smallest part of the extracellular fluids, and the portion content is within the epithelial-lined spaces, where most of the total body water is confined. The primary function of the transcellular fluid is for transportation and lubrication of cavities. Examples include ocular fluid, joint fluid, pleural cavity, and cerebrospinal fluid.

In another definition, transcellular fluid is not regarded among the total body weight of the extracellular fluid; it has a measure of about 2.5% of the total body water.

- **Interstitial fluid**

Interstitial fluid is found in cells with multicellular layers. In order sense, it is not common among simple cells. The fluid occurs in the interstitial spaces or tissue spaces of the cells. Human has multiple layers, and thus increment in interstitial fluid.

The fluid occupies about 11L of the human body and performs a primary function in the transportation of waste and nutrients around the cells. A significant percentage of interstitial fluid performs or acts as the connection between cells and other layers in the body. And the act is seen in a significant function as **interstitial ECM.** The interstitial ECM mainly contains major proteins and connective tissue, through which it transports, aids wound healing, and blood clotting.

- **Blood Plasma**

Blood plasma is the liquid segment of the blood. In it has several dissolved substances, and majorly the blood cells. Aside from the constituted composition, it contains varieties of protein, minerals, nutrients, clotting factors, glucose, globulins, hormones, and the likes.

The major function is transportation, and this is why it has a significant percentage of the blood constitutes—blood plasma is about 55% of the blood volume. However, it contains special blood cells that fight against infections. Furthermore, it aids effective intravascular osmotic measures, whereby the body keeps and maintains the electrolyte levels in the body.

2. **Intracellular Fluid Compartment**

The fluid inside the cells is the intracellular fluid. It is separated into compartments by the membranes that encircle the cells in the body. To better understand the intracellular fluid, it is vital to know the components of a cell.

The cells contain significant components like the nucleus, mitochondria, plastids, and so on. These components are called organelles. In the absence of the organelles, the remaining part of the cell is the cytosol. All organelles are found in the cytosol. Thus, the cytosol is the liquid portion of the cell and the measures of the intracellular fluid of a cell.

The intracellular and extracellular fluids influence processes like signal transduction and osmoregulation. For example, the intracellular fluid contains a low amount of potassium & sodium. This configuration must be maintained so that a necessary process would be carried out effectively.

2.4 Movement of Fluid Between Compartments

Movement by Osmotic Pressure

The main difference between osmotic pressure and hydrostatic pressure is the presence or absence of semipermeable membrane and the difference in concentration of solutes and solvents. Osmotic gradient occurs when the listed factors (semipermeable membrane and concentration of solutes & solvents) are present, unlike hydrostatic pressure. And the magnitude of this gradient is directly proportional to the amount of solute in check—the movement is from a low concentration of solutes to a high concentration of solutes.

The concentration of solutes changes often, and the body adjusts to the change many times in check to balance the water concentration in the body.

A typical example of an osmotic gradient is the movement of water in and out of the body. When a body is covered with sweat, it merely means the organs are losing water, thereby increasing the solutes' concentration in the skin cells. Apparently, the osmotic pressure in the skin cells increases and water begins to flow into the cells' extracellular fluid.

The water movement will cause zero changes in the total body configuration if there is enough water in the body. Conversely, the body will stimulate changes like thirst from the brain as a sign of dehydration if there is a little amount of water in the extracellular fluids.

Mostly, the circle continues like a single thread of water flowing from the blood (around the skin) into the sweat glands and from the glands to the skin tissues that lack water. The amount of water that leaves the blood is extracted from the surrounding fluids, and the circle flows on until the body calls for water—dehydration. On drinking water, the process flows in the same sense, and water is redistributed to the cells that lack or need water to balance their functionality.

Movement by Hydrostatic Pressure

The primary factor contributing to the movement of fluid across the compartments is the force acting on the fluid due to the exerted pressure by the walls of the constituting vessel. For example, hydrostatic pressure has exerted a fluid against the walls of the vessel. And the more the pressure, the more the flow of the fluid. The same pressure is applicable in the movement of blood. Blood pressure is the exertion of force created by the heart while pumping the blood, and thereby the blood flows throughout the body.

On the capillaries, the vessels have high capillary blood pressure compared to the colloid osmotic pressure, and thereby the food nutrients can move out of the capillaries to the body cells that surround the capillaries.
The same principle binds the entering of food nutrients into the capillaries. The capillary blood pressure is lower at the capillaries' venule end, so food nutrients can quickly enter the capillary.

Particularly about the kidney, the hydrostatic pressure of the fluid governs the movement of fluid. When the hydrostatic pressure increases, the amount of water or urine filtration that occurs at the exact moment in time increases. The amount of urine that will pass through the capillaries out into the outside cells increases.

In cases of dehydration or other factors that contribute to low-kidney-function, it means the hydrostatic pressure drops, and the kidney function is pseudo at that moment. Hydrostatic pressure is the main contributor to all kidney functions, even in excretion, detoxification, and filtration.

Movements by Active Transports

Once there is an expenditure of energy, transportation is termed "active transport." Unlike the passive transport of hydrostatic pressure and osmotic pressure, active transport consumes energy in the form of ATP. Active transport is essential when there is a need to move substances against their concentration gradient; that is, the movement of substances from low concentration to a high concentration. Often, the use of special transportation mediums like pumps is required. A typical example is a sodium-potassium pump.

In this case, the movement occurs against the substance's concentration gradient; while potassium is pumped into the cells, sodium is pumped out of the cell.

Another need for a unique transportation system is the nature of the membrane. Often, the membrane layers contain polar factors; thus, non-polar substances will find it difficult to pass through. And therefore, there are various active transport systems for substances like lipids, water, glucose, ions, and amino acids. For example, aquaporins are the water channels in the membrane of the cells that allows water to flow easily into/outside the cells. Another example is the facilitated transport system. This system gives the charge to substances and will enable them to move down a concentration gradient along particular protein passages in the membrane.

2.5 Water Balance

Water balance is the interaction and interpretation of water movement in the body. Water circulation occurs in two stages, which are intake of water circulation and outward circulation. Any deviation between these two makes the body unfit for regular activities. The significance of water balance is the measure of equating all the contents in the body.

For example, a drop of fluid in the body does not contain only water. It has several solutes (substances) dissolved in the fluid. Thus, high or low volume of the fluid in the body will result in specific changes, which may cause several complications in the body.

The regulation of water makes a significant impact in the form of thirst and excretion of water. Channels that are involved in releasing fluids in the body are not limited to one, and thus the rate of excreting waste via fluids is more than the consumption of water.
For example, sweat, urine, breathing, feces, and others are channels through which water leaves the body. Conversely, water intake occurs by direct drinking or administration by serum contents in the form of drips.

Regularly, a healthy person will take 2500mL of water and excrete the same volume per day. The water intake system may vary per person; it might slightly reduce or increase in volume depending on the body's activity. The body adjusts to the level of water demands by the body; on average, the content should be approximately 2500mL. If more is consumed, more of the fluid will be excreted – the significance of homeostasis in the body.

Water balance occurs via the exchange of fluids in the body. A high percentage of water is absorbed or released via the kidney. The kidney contributes more to the regulation of water in the body. Most of the kidney's actions are active-mode; since the body is mostly aware of the action.

For example, a signal is a relay to the brain if less water is absorbed in the kidney, and the human will be thirsty—which is a sign of kidney functionality. In another sense, the kidney releases more water and excretes it as urine when a high percentage of water is consumed. Excretion of water via the urine is also an active-mode of water circling.

Conversely, water loss can occur via evaporation from the skin surfaces. Remember that skin is a sense organ, and one of the functions is water balance. The skin cannot absorb water directly, but water evaporates via the pores on the skin.

Evaporation of water from the skin is insensible water loss because the individual is not aware of any changes during the action. And this is directly the opposite of the active-mode of excreting water from the body.

Either active-water exchange or cold water exchanges the two are essential and able to cause some complications. So, there is a need to know the ways and how water balances in the body—homeostasis.

Homeostasis - The regulation of water intake

The concept of osmolality is used to assess the water balance in the body. By definition, osmolality is the ratio of solute to solvent in a solution. For all fluids, there is specific osmolality at a certain point in time. The state of an individual can be normal, dehydrated, or hypotonic. And this is the reason for all cells to regular water—homeostasis. Several mechanisms are employed to balance out water; some are hormones; others may combine more than one body-system to maintain balance.

Once an individual takes water, the action may not be totally voluntary. The body has several means of requesting hydration, and the medicated one is thirst. More than one activity has occurred before the signs of thirst and other feelings. This is why homeostasis is a broad study of water balance in the body.

When a single drop of water leaves the body, many processes change to adjust to the loss. And this is significant in the aspect of physiological responses.

Osmoreceptors are the sensory part of the hypothalamus, which operates in the thirst center of the gland. Osmoreceptors monitor the level of solutes in the body. When the blood fluid has a high concentration of solutes *(meaning, low amount of water and high osmolality measures),* the hypothalamus receives signals and transmits signals to the brain. The brain transmits signals to the pituitary glands; thus, the surfacing of thirst. This shows the action and reasons for high water consumption when the body feels low or dry mouth. Following the action are the symptoms of dehydration— which are thirst, dry mouth, less activity, low metabolism, and others.

On the hormonal level, the hypothalamus stimulates the release of antidiuretic hormone (ADH), located in the posterior pituitary gland. The discharge causes the kidney to reabsorb water in the formation of urine. In turn, dilute the blood plasma, *which is an action of the (ADH) via the hypothalamus on the kidney.*

Similar action calls for the attention of humans when the body is thirsty. In this sense, the hypothalamus relay message to the sympathetic nervous system, and from SNS to the mouth's salivary gland.

The change causes thick mucus output, low watery mouth, and a decrease in saliva production, dry mouth, and sensation of thirst. The hypothalamus has a significant contribution to the intake of water.

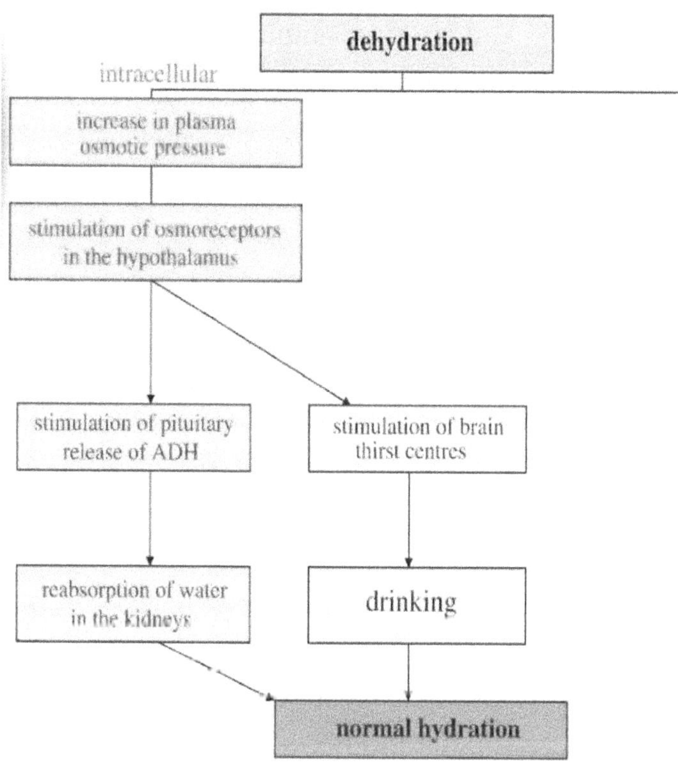

- Water Intake Flowchart

When the volume of blood reduces, the kidneys perform a role in the reabsorption of sodium in the blood. The kidneys have a renin-angiotensin hormonal system that increases the production of hormone angiotensin II. The hormone stimulates the kidney to reabsorb in the distal tubules of the nephrons in the kidneys. In some cases, the circulation of angiotensin II causes the release of ADH.

A decrease in the level of the blood ends in a decrease in blood pressure. And the low amount of blood indicates low blood pressure.

Baroreceptors in the blood, especially at the arch of the aorta and carotid arteries of the neck, detect a decrease in blood pressure. This may not have a direct indication to alert the body system of low water content. However, it is significant to give the heart a signal to pump blood at high pressure to circulate the body.

Homeostasis - The regulation of water output

Loss of water from the body happens prevalently through the renal framework. An individual creates a normal of 15 liters of urine daily. The urine volume differs because of hydration levels; there is a base volume of urine values needed for legitimate substantial capacities.

The kidney discharges 100 to 1200 milliosmoles of solutes to free the body of an assortment of overabundance salts and another water-solvent compound squanders, most remarkably creatinine, uric corrosive, and urea. The inability to deliver the base volume of urine implies metabolic waste cannot be viably taken out from the body, a circumstance that can impede organ work. The base degree of urine creation important to keep up typical capacity is about 0.47 liters each day.

The kidneys additionally should make changes in the case of ingesting a lot of liquid. Diuresis, the production of urine in the abundance of ordinary levels, starts around 30 minutes in the wake of drinking an enormous amount of liquid. Diuresis arrives at its top after approximately 60 minutes, and typical urine production is restored after around 3 hours.

Contribution of Nitrogenous Waste to Water balance

The nitrogen cycle has significance in water balance. Humans are one of the urea-producing mammals, and the excretion has some changes directly associated with water flow. Urea is vital in the metabolism of nitrogenous material in the body. And urea is the main product of nitrogenous waste in humans. The body makes use of urea, and the constitution is non-toxic. However, the body recognizes its high or low volume in the body and initiates an excretion process to balance the product. Urea dissolves in water, with a pH in the neutral range.

During the formation of urine, urea plays an essential role in maintaining water reabsorption or excretion. The flow of urea allows the kidney to detect a low amount of urea, which ultimately calls for reabsorption of water during urine formation. When the body is deficient in water, the urea and high concentration of dissolved substances in the body stimulates the anti-diuretic hormone in the pituitary hormone to initiates the reabsorption of urine in the kidney.

Remember that a high amount of solutes results in an inflow of water by osmosis—in this case, hyperosmotic urine is high in dissolved solutes and solvents; *that is, urine.* On the other hand, hypoosmotic urine is low in dissolved solutes and shows a significant release of more water via the urine channel. *The importance of hyperosmotic and hypoosmotic urine gives the body an average balance in blood pressure, prevents excessive water loss, and maintains a good balance of sodium ions in the blood plasma.*

The significance of the urea cycle is the contribution to water input and water output—homeostasis.

Aldosterone Feedback

Aldosterone is a steroid chemical (corticoid) created toward the finish of the renin-angiotensin framework. To survey the renin-angiotensin structure, low blood volume actuates the juxtaglomerular in an assortment of approaches to discharge renin. Renin cuts angiotensin I from the liver created angiotensinogen. Angiotensin changing over chemical (ACE) in the lungs changes over angiotensin I into angiotensin II. Angiotensin II has an assortment of impacts (like expanding thirst); however, it likewise causes the arrival of aldosterone from the adrenal cortex.

Aldosterone expands water reabsorption; it includes a trade of sodium and potassium that the ADH reabsorption guideline does not have. Aldosterone will likewise cause a comparative particle adjusting effect in the colon and salivary organs.

Aldosterone has various impacts that engaged with the guideline of water yield. It follows up on mineral corticoid receptors in the epithelial cells of the distal tangled tubule and gathering conduit to build their demeanor of Na^+/K^+ ATPase channels and to actuate those channels. This causes extraordinarily expanded reabsorption of sodium and water (which follows sodium osmotically by co-transport) while pushing potassium discharge into the urine.

2.6 Water Balance Disorders

Water balance disorders are common in humans. The causes are many; some are easily traceable, while others are not. The best practice is to know the cause of each change in the water level. The most contributing to water balance disorder is the concept of dehydration and hypovolemia.

On average, dehydration due to water balance disorder is commonly seen in some patients. This is different from the thirst for water due to the low amount of water in the body system. The concept of dehydration resulting from water balance disorders is due to solutes imbalance in the body. *For better understanding, the meaning of hyper-concentration and hypo-concentration of solute in solutions should be well understood.*

Hypovolemia is different from dehydration, although they both contribute to a water balance disorder. By definition, hypovolemia is the reduction in the amount of water in the body due to the decrease in the amount of total blood counts in the body. Hypovolemia is based explicitly on the blood level in the body; it affects the body.

Dehydration

The high content of electrolytes (solutes) in the body leads to a hypertonic solution. This state is characterized by loss of water in the body and ultimately means increased plasma osmolality. Hypertonic dehydration makes the body weak and reduces the overall metabolism in the body.

In most cases, the body refuses to carry out regular activities, and the same can lead to a high chance of complications.

Hypotonic dehydration is the loss of solutes in the solution. The main solute that contributes to hypotonic dehydration is sodium. When sodium is reduced mainly in the body, the body shows decreased plasma osmolality. Thus, water enters the cell from the extracellular fluid. The dehydration via hypotonic means may cause neurological complications like a seizure, alongside depletion in the intravascular water. The water from the intravascular space may shift into the extravascular space when the body undergoes hypotonic dehydration.

Hypovolemia

Aside from overall fluid in the body, hypovolemia describes the amount of blood in the body. When the level of blood starts to decrease in the blood, hypovolemia is significantly observed. When the circulation of fluids in the body begins to reduce, the body experiences specific changes characterized by hypovolemia shock. *This shock disrupts the flow of fluids and inhibits body metabolism on the started levels.*

For example, the flow of food through the alimentary canal demands enough blood capillaries so that the digested particles can be absorbed into the body cells. However, the body will respond slowly to such metabolism since it has a low body volume to cater to the circulation of substances that are already in the blood. Excessive loss of blood, diarrhea, and hemorrhage are the causes of hypovolemia.

Treatment of minor dehydration	*Minor dehydration can be treated by increasing water intake. The dehydration source must be outlined, first, as a lack of water in the body or loss of solutes in the form of electrolytes.* *When water is taken, it increases the level of total fluid in the blood. That is the plasma level increases. However, the loss of solutes can be compensated by taking the required solutes in the form of fluids or other means. For example, sodium levels can be increased by taking high food that is rich in sodium.*

Treatment for Hypovolemia	*The best treatment for hypovolemia is to know the leading cause of the condition. Then, the resulting issue can be addressed using various medical means.* *The best approach to all issues regarding water imbalance in the body is fluid administration to compensate for the whole amount of fluid loss in the body.*

2.7 Intravenous Fluid

The total fluid in the body is made of about 60% water. The division or constitution of this water varies in composition. Nearly 79% is composed in the muscles, and 73% is in the brain and heart. Meaning, the composition of water in each part of the body differs. At regular intervals, the amount of this water should be maintained and kept at constant regulation.

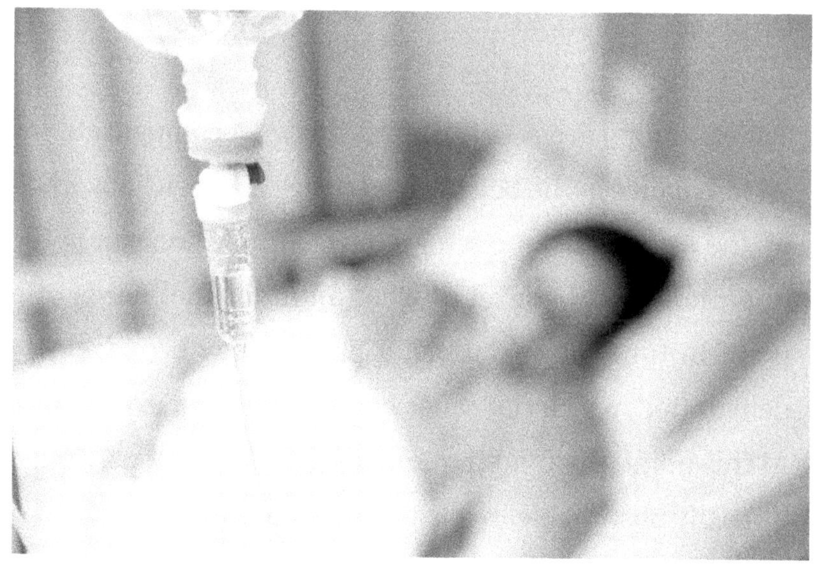

A single loss of water is enough to cause imbalances in the number of electrolytes in the body. When this happens, the kidney reduces its efficiency; the blood becomes thicker, affecting the whole body part; and many differences in activity. All of these features and happening are not evitable; they must occur in the body; as human contribution affects the overall well-being. So the need for intravenous fluids, the administration, and importance in the body. *The mode of administration occurs in two liquid forms, which are crystalloid solutions and colloids. Each of these has uniqueness in handling and the time to use one.*

Crystalloid Solutions

The solutions are administered fluids to compensate for an imbalance in the body because they are easily absorbed by the cells and can circulate fast. Another reason is the importance of the level of what an individual needs at a point in time. For example, a patient may be extremely dehydrated, which can cause complications or even death. At this point, the fluid that must serve intravenously must be easily absorbable in all senses.

The three types of crystalloid solutions vary according to their tonicity—the amount of solute that is present in a solution of a substance.

Crystalloid solutions based on tonicity	
Hypertonic	*The crystalloid solution has more solutes, and therefore more concentrated than the cells. Thus, water flows according to the concentration gradient—that is, out of the cells. The hypertonic crystalloid solution is introduced into the body when the body has more than the required amount of water in the cells.*
Hypotonic	*This solution's osmolality is low, water flows into the cells, unlike the hypertonic solution. More often, solutions like these are introduced into the body when the cell is losing a lot of water. The need for water balance must be compensated.*

Isotonic	*The introduction of isotonic fluids does not cause an increase or decrease in the cell content or extracellular fluids.* *Solutions that are not necessarily prepared for fluid balance are prepared in isotonic form. However, certain levels of this solution must be introduced into the body. This means the introduction of isotonic fluids remains in the target compartments of the body.*

Common intravenous fluids and their administration

The broad grouping is the hypertonic, hypotonic, and isotonic fluids in the intravenous fluids. However, four powerful solutions are immediately administered to maintain stable water balance and regulations in the body.

Crystalloid Solutions	Description and Administration
Lactated Ringers	*This solution maintains the balanced state of the blood plasma concentration. That means it does not affect the blood activities when it is administered to the blood system. The constitution includes potassium chloride, calcium chloride, sodium lactate, and sodium chloride. It is in the form of crystalloid, which means it can be easily absorbed into the body system. The lactated ringers or RL are prepared in distilled water.* *Administration of RL should not be carried out on patients with a low chance of metabolizing lactate. Lactic acidosis is not compatible with lactated ringers, and it is not advisable to administer in such patients.*
Normal Saline of 0.9%	*Normal saline is used in the case of hemorrhage, sepsis, hypovolemia, and dehydration. The composition is prepared in the sterile medium and*

	does not have a significant constitution, just the combination of sodium chloride in pure water. The concentration must be maintained at 0.9% of sodium chloride. *The use of normal saline is applicable in the extracellular fluid. The solution is used in extracellular fluid replacement. And this replacement may count for repletion of loss sodium in the body and treatment and care of metabolic alkalosis in the presence of fluid loss. During an effective treatment, normal saline can be administered to flush the body, especially at the end of the treatment. Flushing the body means the fluid wipes off any waste or accumulation of the*

	earlier-used drugs. Some drugs can cause complications if they are left in the body for a long time. Circulating the normal saline is the best way to address such because the fluid is more like blood plasma; it doesn't cause changes or at least significant changes in the body. Also, the constitutional substances are not more than two—Na & Cl. *The amount of normal saline to be administered varies depending on the age of the patient. An adult may take more volume of saline compared to a young child. Notwithstanding, the weight and nature of the condition must be considered before administration. Thus, the nature of the condition, weight, and age must be*

	observed before the administration. The administration occurs via intravenous (IV) access, and this is the only access. *This fluid is the only one used in line with blood product administration.*
Half Normal Saline (0.45%)	*The half-normal saline is not the same as the 0.9% concentration. The value is hypotonic, and the crystalloid solution permits the water to enter the blood cells. It is ultimately important that the concentration and amount to be administered is a measure to prevent the red blood cells' hemolysis. Half normal saline can ultimately contribute to edema, especially pulmonary edema.* *The solution is administered only when the level of water balance is changing in the body and is only applied in the case and treatment of hypernatremia.*
Dextrose 5% in water	*This solution is different from others mentioned so*

	far. It consists of hypotonic dextrose, which is absorbed by the body. Where the absorption occurs, the cells have enough dextrose concentration, and the remaining fluid (water is isotonic). The dextrose is absorbed by the cells that need the substance. However, the isotonic fluid and its constituted electrolytes remain in the body fluids to keep the intravenous fluids' volume intact and provide water for kidney function. *The solution is not directly used in replenishing the fluid content in the body. This is so as it dilutes the solutes in the fluid when the dextrose is absorbed. The primary purpose is to supply dextrose to the cells and serve as an additional advance of increasing*

	water level in the kidney and cells.

Colloids Solutions

The significant difference from a crystalloid is the solubility and ability to pass through the semipermeable membrane. The colloid particles are too large to pass easily, and thus they are not quickly absorbed by the cells. The significance of this solution is the means of expanding the plasma membrane. The colloid solutions can draw water from the surrounding layers of blood cells into the blood vessels, thereby increasing the plasma level of the blood.

If the body system of a patient cannot tolerate or maintain the standard volume in the plasma, this solution can be administered. Also, it is crucial in patients with malnutrition cases.

Table 3. **Composition of Commercially Available Intravenous Crystalloid Solutions for Fluid Therapy.***

Fluid	Glucose	Sodium	Chloride	Potassium	Buffer†	Calcium	Magnesium	pH	Osmolarity	Osmolality	Electrolyte-free Water
	g/dl	*millimoles per liter*							*mOsm/liter*	*mOsm/kg*	*%‡*
Human plasma	0.07–0.11	135–144	95–105	3.5–5.3	23–30	2.2–2.6	0.8–1.2	7.35–7.45	308	288	0
5% Dextrose in water	5	0	0	0	0	0	0	3.5–6.5	252		100
4% Dextrose in 0.18% saline	4	30	30	0	0	0	0	3.5–6.5	282		81
5% Dextrose in 0.2% saline	5	34	34	0	0	0	0	3.5–6.5	321		78
5% Dextrose in 0.45% saline	5	77	77	0	0	0	0	3.5–6.5	406		50
5% Dextrose Ringer's lactate	5	130	109	4	28	1.5	0	4.0–6.5	525		13
5% Dextrose in 0.9% saline	5	154	154	0	0	0	0	3.5–6.5	560		0
5% Dextrose multiple electrolytes injection, type 1 USP	5	140	98	5	50	0	1.5	4.0–6.5	547		6
Ringer's lactate	0	130	109	4	28	1.35	0	6–7.5	273	254	13
Ringer's acetate	0	130	112	5	27	1	1	6–8	276		12
Hartmann's solution	0	131	111	5	29	2	0	5.0–7.0	278		12
0.9% Saline	0	154	154	0	0	0	0	4.5–7	308	286	0
Multiple electrolytes injection, type 1, USP§	0	140	98	5	50	0	1.5	4.0–6.5	294		6
Isotonic electrolyte solution¶	0	140	127	4	29	2.5	1	4.6–5.4	304		6

* To convert the values for glucose to millimoles per liter, multiply by 0.05551. To convert the values for potassium to milligrams per deciliter, divide by 0.2558. To convert the values for calcium to milligrams per deciliter, divide by 0.250. To convert the values for magnesium to milligrams per deciliter, divide by 0.4114. USP denotes United States Pharmacopeia.
† The buffer is bicarbonate in plasma, lactate in Ringer's lactate and Hartmann's solution, acetate in Ringer's acetate, acetate (27 mmol per liter) and gluconate (23 mmol per liter) in multiple electrolytes injection, type 1, USP, and acetate (23 mmol per liter) and maleate (5 mmol per liter) in isotonic electrolyte solution.
‡ This percentage is based on a sodium plus potassium concentration in the aqueous phase of plasma of 154 mmol per liter, assuming that plasma is 93% water with a plasma sodium concentration of 140 mmol per liter and a potassium concentration of 4 mmol per liter.
§ Multiple electrolytes injection, type 1, USP, is the generic name for Plasma-Lyte 148, Normosol, and Isolyte.
¶ Isotonic electrolyte solution is the generic name for Sterofundin and Ringerfundin. It has an electrolyte composition that is similar to that of plasma.

Colloids solutions are not common, like crystalloid. However, they are essential. The administration of this solution is common in cases like peritonitis, shock, and external burns. Because water is reduced naturally from the plasma, the solution can supply water for effective circulation.

Intravenous Therapy

Intravenous treatment (condensed as IV treatment) is a clinical strategy that conveys liquids and nourishment straightforwardly into an individual's vein.

The intravenous course of the organization is ordinarily utilized for rehydration or to give sustenance to individuals who can't burn through food or water by mouth.

It might likewise be used to regulate meds or other clinical treatments, for example, blood items or electrolytes, to address lopsided electrolyte characteristics.

Efforts to give intravenous therapy have been recorded as right on time as the 1400s.

However, the training did not get inescapable until the 1900s after advancing strategies

for protected, practical use.

The intravenous course is the quickest method to convey meds and fluids substitution through the body. They are brought straightforwardly into the circulatory structure and immediately dispersed along these lines. Thus, the intravenous course of organization is additionally utilized for the utilization of some sporting medications.

Numerous treatments are managed as a "bolus" or a one-time portion, yet they may likewise be controlled as all-inclusive implantation. The demonstration of controlling a treatment intravenously, or putting an intravenous line ("IV line") for some time in the future, is a technique that should just be performed by a gifted proficient.

The essential intravenous access comprises a needle penetrating the skin and entering a vein associated with a needle or outer tubing. This is utilized to control the ideal treatment in situations where a patient is probably going to get numerous such intercessions in a brief period (with an ensuing danger of injury to the vein). The typical practice is to embed a cannula that leaves one end in the vein, and resulting treatments can be directed effectively through tubing at the opposite end. At times, different meds or treatments are controlled through a similar IV line.

IV lines are delegated "focal lines" In the event that they end in a huge vein near the heart or as "fringe lines" if their yield is to a little vein in the outskirts, like the arm. An IV line can be strung through a fringe vein to end close to the heart, named an "incidentally embedded focal catheter" or PICC line. Suppose an individual is probably going to require long-haul intravenous treatment. In that case, a clinical port might be embedded to empower simpler rehashed admittance to the vein without puncturing the vein consistently. A catheter can likewise be implanted into a focal vein through the chest, known as a burrowed line.

The particular sort of catheter utilized and site of addition are influenced by the ideal substance to be managed and the veins' soundness in the perfect inclusion site.

Arrangement of an IV line may cause torment, as it essentially includes penetrating the skin. Diseases and irritation (named phlebitis) are additionally both regular results of an IV line. Phlebitis might be almost inevitable if a similar vein is utilized consistently for intravenous access and can ultimately form into a hard rope which is unsatisfactory for IV access. The accidental organization of treatment outside a vein, named extravasation or penetration, may cause opposite results.

2.8 Water Volume Regulation and Volume Overload

Water volume and chronic diseases

The significance of extracellular fluid volume is used in the explanation of the water volume in the body. The overall expansion of this ECF is the water volume, that is, the wide circulation of the fluid per specific location in the body. While some parts may have a low amount of fluids, overload may occur in other locations due to underlying causes. Most overload conditions are due to chronic diseases. An exception is simple imbalances of solutes in the body which was described as primary renal retention.

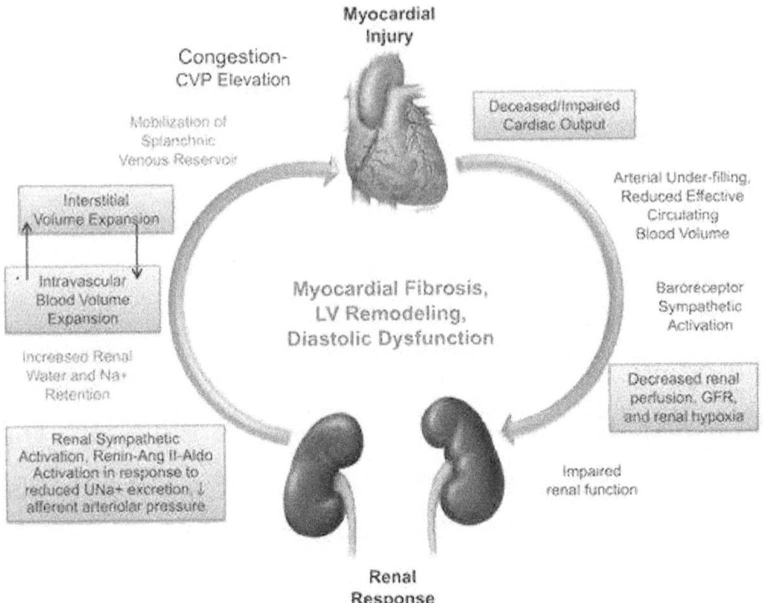

The activation of the aldosterone system in cirrhosis of the liver leads to splanchnic vasodilation and typically accumulates more water, resulting in ascites and edema. The significant trigger here is the retention of renal salts and water.

Apart from the time a patient is administered with several loads of fluids as intravenous fluids, the most commonly suitable for excessive extracellular fluids are due to the liver's cirrhosis, heart failure, and other chronic diseases. Some drawbacks compensate heart failure in the amount of solute that is directly present in the cells.

A high amount of these salts draws in water from the surrounding fluids and increases the water content; the activation of aldosterone largely influences this, and thus an approach to reduce the cardiac output towards normal by increasing the preload.

Water volume regulation and medical cases

Volume overload is due to several causes, and the significant one is the retention of salt or other solutes. After a laboratory test, if the cause is confirmed to be an issue of salt retention, the approach will be as primary or secondary causes. Salt retention has effects as the main cause of volume overload (primary cause) or secondary cause. The signs of aldosteronism are observed when the primary cause by salt retention. That is, the volume overload is directly due to hypertension causes, as the case may be.

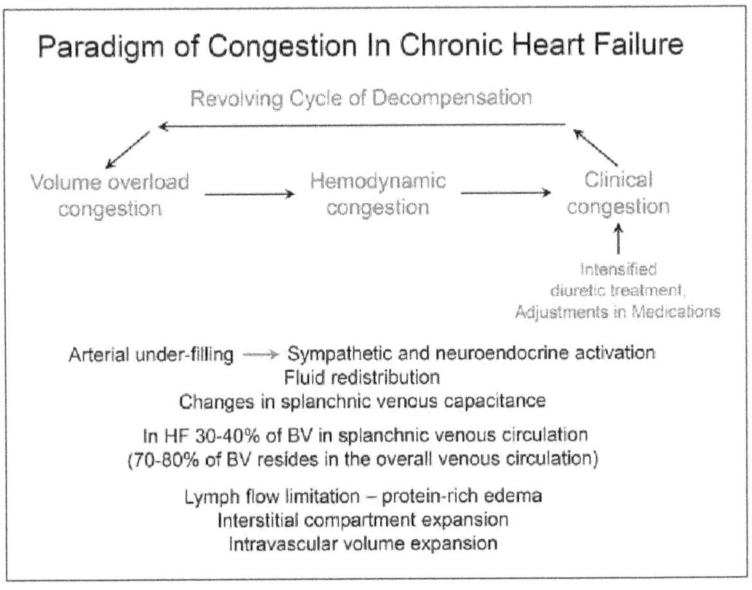

On the other hand, the secondary causes of volume overload regarding salt retention must have an underlying cause. Meaning, the salt would only be retained (which causes volume overload) if the underlying cause persists. Thus, the best medical approach to volume overload is to know the leading cause of the condition and to classify the water volume as "primary or secondary renal salt retention."

Nephrotic syndrome is another chronic disease that contributes to high volume overload in a patient. The syndrome is analyzed by the presence of edema, hyperlipidemia, hypoalbuminemia, proteinuria with less than 3.5 grams/day, and thrombosis as an additional feature.

Nephrotic syndrome is analyzed into three, depending on the type and location.

- *Nephritic process and a typical example post-infectious glomerulonephritis*
- *Bland nephropathy as in the case of minimal change disease*
- *A sclerotic process is characterized by segmental abs focal glomerulonephritis.*

Edema, dyspnea, fatigue, and abdominal distention are signs of volume overload. The central importance of these symptoms is the sense of identifying the cause of the problem. Another implication is the use as an identifier in underlying causes and the symptoms. For example, typical edema might become worse (via excessive swells up) after a few hours.

Furthermore, dyspnea is characterized by heart failure if the condition grows beyond measures. Jaundice and dark urine are signs of cirrhosis which is a good sign in identifying the causes and suitable
treatments.

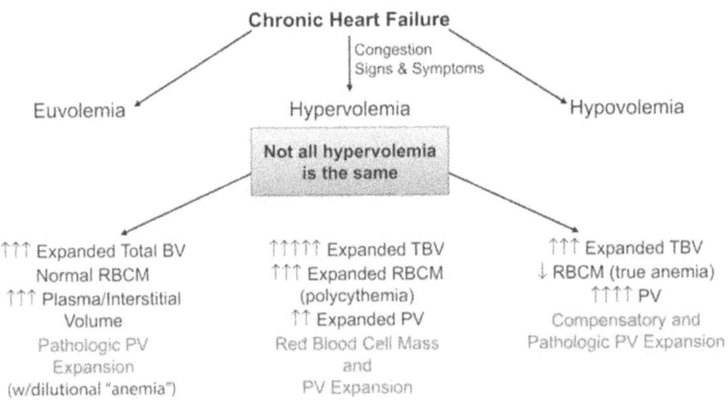

Another thing is the underlying causes of volume overload. As mentioned earlier, a volume overload sign does not necessarily show a direct collaboration between the volume overload and a fixed cause. For example, an indication of systolic dysfunction will result in low blood pressure and volume overload symptoms. For an excellent treatment, volume overload is not the primary goal here; it's a predominant pedal for systolic dysfunction in the heart. Also, in cirrhosis, the blood pressure becomes low as a result of systemic vasodilation.

It is different from systolic dysfunction, as this is directly related to the hyper-dynamic circulation of fluid in the body system. The determinant is mostly seen as the accumulation of fluids in the body's abdominal cavity, although edema may be present in some cases.

Aside from the chronic causes of volume overload in the body, the amount of renal salt and retention also contributes to volume overload. When the body fluid is low, there is renal perfusion reduction which thus increases salt retention. The presence of proteinuria may continue to stimulate the reabsorption of renal salts. This can further stimulate the active transport of the sodium channels in the cells of the distal nephron. More impairs to sodium balance in the kidney can quickly promote a considerable accumulation of water, and the effect is mostly felt as peripheral edema or other conditions.

Chapter 3

3.0 Serum Potassium

Potassium ion is plenteous in the body and mainly accumulates in its intracellular components compared to the extracellular fluid. While serum sodium concentration is independent of sex, the concentration is high in males and preferably low in females and old patients. Also, the concentration of serum potassium should be maintained at the range of 3.5 to 5.5 mEq/L. However, the amount of this substance is high or average in many parts of the body. It is relatively low in the plasma.

The division of serum potassium varies across all the body cells. It is high in the intracellular fluids and low in the extracellular fluids. Likewise, the total composition of serum potassium is about 55 mEq/kg of a typical body. Of all these compositions, the skin muscle and subcutaneous tissue take 98% of the total composition, leaving the extracellular compartments with the remaining 2%. Standard functionality of cells is widely contributed by the action of serum potassium on the particular cell.

Meaning, potassium equivalent in the extracellular and intracellular fluids must be maintained at some values. Thus, (K_e: K_i) shows cells' formation, either active or has less contribution to the body. Another significance of the ratio is the determinant of resting membrane potential in a cell. All of these are Na-K-ATPase factors, directly influencing the flow of potassium and sodium in the cells.

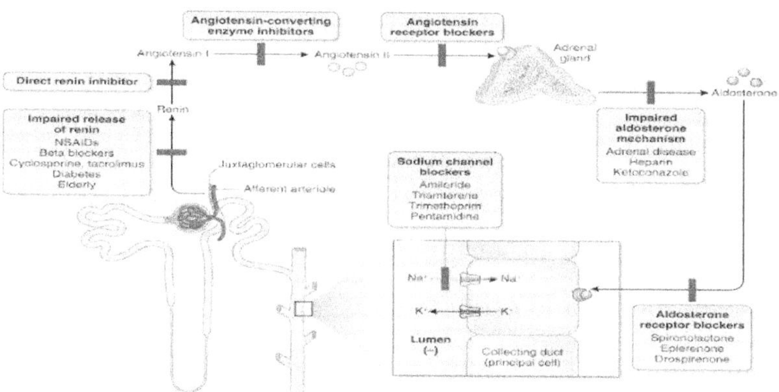

Humans are exposed to high potassium consumption in most of their diets; the effect on the body differs based on the consumption rate. Likewise, potassium deficiency is not commonly observed in patients that eat healthily. The average amount of potassium in the body should not exceed 100 mEq/day on normal conditions. The intake of potassium from foods may vastly be increased or decreased depending on the inflow. If the concentration is higher than 100 mEq/day, it is considered a high-amount of serum potassium.

The influx dictates how the kidney flushes out potassium or how it retains it. When the concentration is high, the kidney removes the high amount of potassium from the body. When the concentration is low, the kidney maintains the potassium amount in the body by reabsorbing potassium.

If the case of high/low potassium, which directly changes (Ke: Ki), when the body adjusts to the change because the ratio is significant to cause some complications if it is not solved quickly. Potassium is directly related to body cell formation/functionality and also the resting potential. Thus, the action of serum potassium contributes to the muscles, bone, and other tissues.

When the (K_e: K_i) favors the intracellular compartment; that is, the compartment increases compare to the extracellular compartment; the kidney moves potassium ions into the intracellular of some other cells, and directly balance the ratio until the kidney can resolve the issues, via the action of hormones and other secretions.

In summary, acidemia and an increase in a cell's osmolality move potassium ions out of the cell. Conversely, aldosterone, insulin, alkalemia, and catecholamines directly stimulate potassium ions into the cell.

Insulin is a hormone that functions in moving potassium out of the cell (reducing serum potassium) into the muscles and liver. The main contributor to insulin production is the high level of serum potassium. When the fluid is higher than the required amount in a specific body location, insulin acts by converting the potassium into serum potassium in the liver and muscles. Unlike insulin, catecholamines act by influencing beta-2 receptors to move potassium out of a cell—performing the same insulin function. Aside from the regulation of potassium via the secretion of insulin and catecholamines, the two factors can be administered and cause significant changes in the body's level of potassium.

In the balance of serum potassium, acid-base balance and plasma osmolality do not perform like their well-known features; the two contribute to balance in serum potassium. Acid-base is significant in moving potassium into the cell when the concentration of H^+ changes. Specifically, the body sense changes in the amount of H^+ when the amount of ion reduces; the body takes in potassium ions instead.

Conversely, during an acidemia, the movement of potassium is out of the cell. Lastly, osmolality also moves potassium out of the cell by moving water when there is a sudden increase in a cell's osmolality.

The major contributor to the balance in potassium in the body is the kidney. The kidney does not take in a small amount of potassium, unlike the earlier mentioned factors. The kidney reabsorbs about 90% of potassium and equally distributes the substance to balance all features in the body. Note, the reabsorbed potassium from the kidney is different from the final urinary potassium after the last cycle. The distal convoluted and outer medullary collecting tubules largely contribute to the excretion of potassium in a cell. Unlike the other factors like serum potassium, the urinary potassium cannot be absorbed to the least value. When there is a low amount of serum potassium, the collecting tubules changes function and reabsorb the urinary potassium, but not all percentage. Thus, there will always be some potassium values in the blood—about 10 - 15 mEq/day. Factors like urine flow rate, potassium intake, intracellular potassium concentration, distal amount of sodium, and mineralocorticoid activity contribute to the rate of potassium excretion in the body.

Clinical significance of serum potassium

Clinical mortality and morbidity are associated with a slight decrease in the amount of potassium serum. The features can surface even at slight changes in the concentration with less than 1.0 mEq/L. Thus, the normal range of sodium-potassium should be at the range of 3.5 - 5.5 mEq/L.

The treatment of the high or low amount of serum potassium is critical. This is because changes in serum potassium are able to cause complications in the body. For example, a slight reduction or increase of about 1.0 mEq/L can increase/reduce the (K_e: K_i) by 25%. And this is enough to stop significant changes and processes in the body.

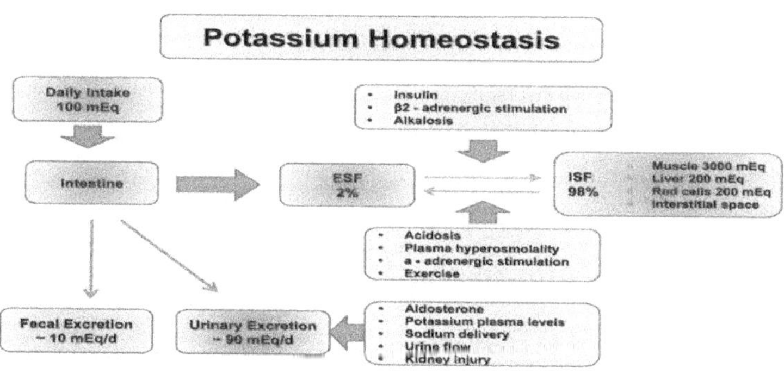

Hypokalemia

Hypokalemia cannot be deduced from the total amount of serum potassium because it can coexist with a deficiency or high serum potassium percentage. When the body excretes more urinary potassium, the significance may not be noticed in the serum potassium. And this affects the classification as either hypokalemia or hyperkalemia.

Hypokalemia may occur when the total body potassium is normal. When this happens, it merely shows that more potassium is absorbed into the cells, maybe by the action of high exogenous or endogenous catecholamines or insulins. The main cause of hypokalemia is the presence of alkalemia, as explained earlier.
Alkalemia may change in the metabolic or respiratory origin, and the change in pH may be used to adjust and correct the amount of potassium value in the body.

The total body potassium can also be used to measure the amount of potassium in the body. The difference from hypokalemia caused by alkalemia is that this is due to a deficiency in the body's potassium. When the deficit is traced, it can be grouped as 1.0 mEq/L deficiency or 2.0 mEq/L; the initial follows that 200 to 300 mEq reduce in serum potassium, and the latter shows 500 to 600 mEq deficit in the total body potassium. A single change in potassium may not show the cause and the right values of total body potassium. To access these values and ascertain that the measure concerning the potassium is normal, several things like the patient's medical history, laboratory tests, and other factors must be considered.

The deficiency of potassium in total body count is directly due to potassium loss as urinary potassium or low potassium consumption. The deficiency due to insufficient consumption is not commonly observed. However, a patient may easily pass more than the required amount of potassium through the urinary tracts. The only way to see a patient suffering from potassium deficiency due to reduced consumption may be due to loss-weight programs.

The loss of potassium as urinary potassium is not common. Typically, the amount of potassium in the urine is quantified, which means the presence of potassium in the urine means that it is to be excreted. However, impaired urinary tracts may develop a loss of potassium mechanism than normal.

The urinary potassium is conserved as a proper sense or signal when the urinary tubules absorb some percentage due to the low amount of potassium in the body.

Notwithstanding, the urinary potassium is more excreted when the disordered urinary tract stimulates the production of aldosterone. More aldosterone signifies high dehydration and urine formation, and more urine leads to increased loss of urinary potassium. This is a common and straightforward way by which the urinary potassium is lost in excess. The body quickly tends to be in hypokalemia due to this cause.

Aside from those potassium losses, the loss of potassium can occur as renal potassium loss. And this is commonly associated with a high level of aldosterone. Conditions like hypochloremia, metabolic alkalosis, and increased urine level are causes of renal potassium wastage. And this occurs as diuretics that include kaliuresis through several mechanisms. Other reasons for renal potassium waste are due to the primary increase in the circulation of mineralocorticoids.

Hyperkalemia

Serum potassium above 5.5 mEq/L ought to be animated quickly and treated with care. Serum potassium above 6.5 mEq/L is related to critical horribleness and mortality and ought to be taken care of as a crisis.

Arrangement of hyperkalemia is into three: pseudohyperkalemia, hyperkalemia with typical complete body potassium, and hyperkalemia with high absolute body potassium.

Pseudohyperkalemia connotes an in vitro (i.e., the in vivo serum potassium is typical). This is brought about by the arrival of potassium from cell parts of blood during the way toward coagulating and, less generally, by the arrival of potassium from ischemic muscle cells because of a tight hand/arm practice during the blood-drawing measure.

If hyperkalemia with high absolute body potassium is suspected, blood should flow appropriately again, and serum potassium lessens in the body. If the previous is presumed, the platelet and white cell collaboration should be checked, and serum should be reviewed for huge hemolysis.

Hyperkalemia happens when there is thrombocytosis (platelet tally more noteworthy than 600,000), leukocytosis (WBC more prominent than 200,000), or huge hemolysis (serum hemoglobin more noteworthy than 1.5 g/dl). If thrombocytosis or serious leukocytosis is available, plasma potassium should be estimated.

On the basis that the hemolysis level is known, blood draw should be deliberately rehashed.

Hyperkalemia with typical absolute body potassium is brought about by the move of potassium out of the cell. It is usually found in acidemia, abrupt expansion in plasma osmolality, huge tissue breakdown, extremely uncommon conditions, adrenergic blockage, and hyperkalemic intermittent loss of motion.

Acidemia is, by a long shot, the primary source of hyperkalemia. As shown, mineral acidosis (e.g., renal disappointment acidosis) is related to the moves in (1.0 mEq/L for each 0.1 U diminishing in pH) of potassium. However, natural acidosis (e.g., lactic acidosis) is related to the uncommon chance of having hyperkalemia. Respiratory acidosis brings about an unobtrusive move (0.2 mEq/L for each 0.1 pH change). These figures, while inexact, can be utilized to address the deliberate serum potassium. Beta barricade can bring about huge hyperkalemia during and following the activity. This is because the potassium at first delivered from the muscle cells is typically taken up by these cells through the incitement of beta-2 receptors by catecholamines.

An unexpected ascent in osmolality can bring about a hidden expansion in serum potassium (0.3 to 0.5 mEq/L); this ascent, in any case, can be a lot more prominent in diabetic patients, who need regular insulin and aldosterone reactions to hyperkalemia.

Hyperkalemia with increment in total body potassium is quite often brought about by reducing potassium's renal discharge. It is infrequently the consequence of an expansion in admission alone. Patients with ordinary kidney capacity can adjust to increment in potassium admission except if the potassium is given quickly (e.g., intravenous implantation) or is given to a patient with a renal imperfection in potassium discharge.

A decrease in renal potassium discharge is either essential renal in the beginning or brought about by a deformity in the renin-angiotensin-aldosterone layer. Although potassium discharge is essentially a secretory change, constant diminishes in glomerular filtration rate (GFR) to under 20 ml/min can be related to hyperkalemia.

In patients with generally ordinary GFR, hyperkalemia is typical because of a deformity in the renin-angiotensin-aldosterone layer or to an imperfection in the rounded renal responsiveness to aldosterone. In these patients, estimation of plasma aldosterone level and, if necessary, further assessment of the renin-angiotensin-aldosterone pivot might be needed for authoritative determination.

Chapter 4

4.0 Serum Phosphate

The concentration of serum phosphate is best expressed in milligrams per deciliter. This best represents the concentration in millimoles which is not static in a factor-like acid-base status. The amount and level of serum phosphate are not the same in the body. Serum phosphate is widely used and transported across the body. In the serum form, the phosphate is in two forms: *mono-hydrogen phosphate and dihydrogen phosphate.* The balanced relationship between the mono and dihydrogen phosphate is calculated or seen via the Henderson-Hasselbalch equation. The equation shows the significances of this serum at both the physiological level and the conversion importance. For example, at the physiological ends, the ratio between the dihydrogen and monohydrogen phosphate is 4:1, and the pH level of the same substance is relatively at a neutral level of 7.40.

The amount of serum phosphate varies per individual. Moreover, the range is between 3.4 - 4.5 mg/dl. The substance is an age-based function.

It differs in concentration per individual (age); it is high in young children compared to an adult. Also, it is commonly increased via dietary intake, such that the diurnal variation reaches its nadir between 8 - 11 am.

Phosphate is a significant intracellular substance in the intracellular of humans, and it is widely distributed across all the cells. Most of the percentage is in the skeleton of hydroxyapatite and relatively low in soft tissues. Phosphate is found more in a person with high body weight (or body composition) and alternatively low in an individual with less body composition. The phosphate level in the extracellular fluid can measure the body status and reactions to specific changes.

Also, phosphate in the extracellular fluids is in the composition of *inorganic phosphate,* which is relatively low compared to the intracellular phosphate, and the composition is also different. Since the extracellular fluid contains inorganic phosphate, then; most of the body phosphate is in inorganic form. And they cover the lipids, carbohydrates, and proteins alongside all these substances, the inorganic phosphate combined with them to form varieties of organic composition and perform changes in the body.

The phosphate's specific functionality contributes to the formation of various organic-organizations, including mitochondria, cytoplasm, and cell structure (walls and other compartments). Another function is forming certain enzymes, stimulating different enzymes, and other activities in processes like glycolysis. In glycolysis, phosphate performs several enzymatic processes.

Phosphate is found in composition like ammonia genesis and also in the oxidative phosphorylation of certain substances. And lastly, the energy from the formation of adenosine diphosphate to adenosine triphosphate. The serum phosphate also affects the regulation of 2,3-diphosphoglycerate synthesis, and in turn, contributes to the action of hemoglobin in carrying oxygen effectively.

- **Test for serum phosphate**

  This test is carried out specifically by using a means analyzed as isotopic or colorimetrical methods. The use of Sub-barow and Fiske techniques is a widely used mode of executing the colorimctrical method of testing serum phosphate. At first, the technique of colorimetrical focuses on the formation of phosphomolybdic acid at the beginning of the process.

Then, phosphomolybdic acid is reduced to molybdenum which is blue in classification, using stannous chloride.

The confirmation of phosphate in the body may be affected by proteins, carbohydrates, and other substances in the body. Thus, molybdenum formation is carried out alongside several other processes to outline the serum level in the body. This is crucial to excellent living and prevents slight medical complications.

Before the test, the serum phosphate should be maintained at the proper level by fasting. A fasting patient maintains a certain phosphate level, which is the main result needed by the test.
Other activities like a recent meal, muscular and hyperventilate actions may reduce the amount of phosphate in the blood.

The body does not lose phosphate easily, as it is prevalent in daily foods. On a single consumption, an individual takes in about 1.0 - 1.5 g/day of phosphorus. About 75 - 80% are absorbed into the digestive system cells involved in the breakdown of the substance; the rest is excreted via the same canal.

A high consumption rate implies a high absorption rate. However, the alimentary canal compensates for the excess consumption by eliminating some values from the total consumption. Likewise, low consumption of phosphorus implies a complete absorption by the alimentary canal. While the extra percentage is somehow compensated for, the low consumption rate is very easy to have all-absorbed values.

At the cellular level, the absorption of phosphorus in the body occurs via the passive diffusion of the substance between cells and more contributed by the size and type of cells involved. On the other hand, the assimilation of phosphorus into the body system is via active transport, which is fast and most effective. In the alimentary canal, after the consumption of phosphorus, it is more absorbed by luminal cells' action, more importantly, via intraluminal sodium, that is, the presence or absence of sodium at this level affects the absorption of phosphorus in the body. The fundamental parts of a digestive intestine may absorb phosphorus, more importantly via the action of the jejunum, then duodenum, and ileum. While all these absorb serum phosphate directly, the absorption via jejunal is vitamin D dependant.
The effective absorption of this substance is mainly due to the presence or absence of vitamin D.

The kidney contributes to significant changes observed in serum phosphate since it is the central organ that monitors and excretes phosphate waste from the body. On absorption of phosphorus into the body system, especially at the plasma level, the kidney ultra-filtrates about 80% of the plasma protein. Conversely, filtrates of about 85 - 90% of phosphate are absorbed by the kidney. The absorption of phosphate is mostly dependent on the level of phosphorus in the body. A high amount of phosphate gives a relatively mild contribution to kidney reabsorption. And low consumption or presence of phosphorus in the body leads to wide reabsorption of phosphate in the body. In the kidney, the reabsorption occurs via the proximal tubules, and this is where the major reabsorption occurs. Note that the reabsorption of this substance is not homogeneous—the proximal tubules first absorb a large concentration or components of the substance. Then the remaining portion is absorbed in other parts of the proximal tubules.

Hypophosphatemia

The term signifies serum concentration of phosphate that is lower than 2.5 mg/dl. Although a patient with less than 1 mg/dl is observed, which is commonly symptomatic, such levels are often labeled as severe hypophosphatemia.

Most phosphate deficiencies occur via a reduction in the total body phosphorus; however, the term hypophosphatemia does not necessarily result from a reduction in the total body phosphorus.
Most of the condition that leads to hypophosphatemia includes glucose ingestion, low dietary intake ECV expansion, respiratory alkalosis, and insulin administration.

The three central breakdowns of hypophosphatemia are observed in three levels which are:

- Low intake of dietary that is rich in phosphorus
- The transcellular shift of phosphorus from the extracellular fluids to surrounding cells
- Increased phosphate excretion from the body.

The loss of phosphorus which is not related to renal failure occurs in the gut. This is typically linked to malabsorption which might be as a result of certain conditions like diarrheal. Also, deficiency in vitamin D in children is able to cause phosphorus deficiency because of a poor absorption rate of the substance. Lastly the phosphate binders may not bind with selected phosphate at the cellular level, but bind with other substances with the same configuration as a typical phosphate.

Significant changes in phosphorus can happen through the kidneys. The typical reason for renal phosphate changes is the abundance of parathyroid chemicals, which decreases the most extreme renal rounded reabsorption of phosphorus. These imperfections might be innate or gained. Among the innate deformities, the most popular is Fanconi's condition—a proximal cylindrical problem creating phosphaturia, glycosuria, aminoaciduria, uricosuria, and bicarbonaturia.

A comparative picture may likewise be seen in cystinosis, Wilson's sickness, innate fructose prejudice, and glycogen stockpiling infection. Procured deserts incorporate numerous myeloma, amyloidosis, and weighty metal inebriation. In post renal transplantation, a condition of optional hyperparathyroidism may exist, with high coursing parathyroid chemical bringing about phosphate squandering by ordinary renal tubules. Such a state may persevere for a while.

Nutrient D-safe rickets is accepted to be brought about by a phosphate spill from renal tubules alongside uncommon intestinal assimilation of phosphate.

Renal rounded squandering can likewise happen during extracellular volume extension with saline or bicarbonate.

Such an image can be seen during the diuretic period of intense cylindrical putrefaction or with the utilization of diuretic specialists.

Treatment

The treatment of hypophosphatemia includes detecting the reason and rectifying the hidden condition. Phosphate supplementation is not needed for mild to direct asymptomatic hypophosphatemia.

In any case, serious hypophosphatemia (under 1.0 mg/dl) or suggestive hypophosphatemia requires quick adjustment. Phosphate can be supplanted by one or the other oral or parenteral organization. Like potassium, phosphate substitution treatment is empiric in light of the fact that total body phosphorus is not resolved without any problem. Occasional checking of the serum phosphate is needed during substitution treatment.

Hyperphosphatemia

Hyperphosphatemia happens in a few endocrine conditions related to expanded rounded reabsorption of phosphate. In pseudohypoparathyroidism, there is a shortage of parathyroid chemicals to follow up on renal tubules, bringing about a high "Tm," which is answerable for the high serum phosphate within sight of an unusual coursing parathyroid chemical.

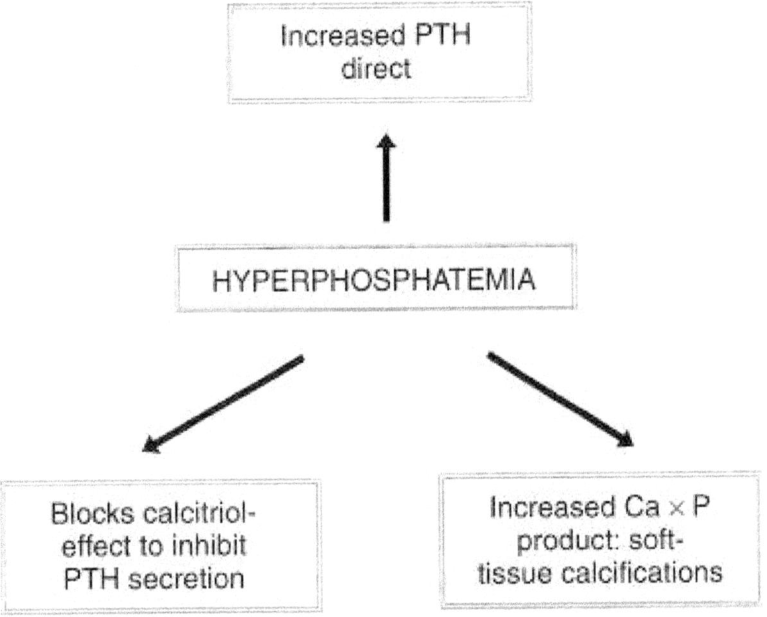

In acromegaly, overabundance in development chemicals prompts expanded cylindrical reabsorption of phosphate. In other clinical circumstances with a high serum phosphate, there is expanded reabsorption of phosphate.

Consequently, in deficient magnesium, there is diminished arrival of parathyroid chemicals, creating scene-like hypoparathyroidism.

In tumoral calcinosis, a condition seen all the more regularly in blacks, there has all the earmarks of being essential expanded reabsorption of phosphate with regular GI ingestion of calcium. With the organization of nutrient D or its analogs, there is expanded ingestion of calcium and phosphate from the gastrointestinal plot; if there is some level of renal inadequacy, hyperphosphatemia may result.

The symptomatology of hyperphosphatemia is identified with the conditions delivering it. The most widely recognized danger is ectopic or metastatic calcification, which may happen if the result of the serum calcium and phosphorus surpasses 70. The calcification may happen in any organ, despite the fact that it is seen most normally in the cornea, conjunctiva, lungs, and skin. Calcification is encouraged by alkalosis. Vascular calcification can deliver gangrene just as it stores in the heart directing structure. Treatment comprises distinguishing the basic reason and rectifying it.

In renal deficiency, treatment comprises controlling dietary admission of phosphates and utilization of phosphate fasteners. Inception of dialysis helps in controlling serum phosphate levels; however, in itself is once in a while powerful.

The symptomatology of hyperphosphatemia is identified with the conditions creating it. The most well-known danger is ectopic or metastatic calcification, which may happen if the result of the serum calcium and phosphorus.

Chapter 5

5.0 Serum Sodium

The amount of sodium in the body should be in the range of 137mEq/L to 142 mEq/L. Certain body changes cause any deviation from this range. And this is why the serum sodium must be monitored and balanced at all times.

The accumulation of the serum sodium focus is frequently seen in hospitalized patients and may give the clinician significant deductions concerning the nature or seriousness of the fundamental infection measure. It is vital to push the applied significance of recognizing the body sodium content and sodium centralization in body liquids.

Dynamic, energy-requiring measures at the cell limit prohibit sodium from the intracellular compartment and, for viable purposes, keep it to the extracellular fluid. There is the administration of fluids in sodium fixation by expansion or expulsion of water from the extracellular compartment.

Changes in the substance of sodium animate expansion or expulsion of water and accordingly decide the volume of the extracellular liquid.

Two systems serve to keep up the plasma sodium fixation in a tight reach in an individual; they are thirst and antidiuretic chemical (arginine vasopressin) discharge. The convergence of osmotically active plasma solutes, sodium is the most significant, oversees these controls. The commitment of sodium to plasma osmolality is evident from the equation for ascertaining plasma osmolality.

Without hyperglycemia or renal retention, sodium fixation is the lead determinant of plasma osmolality. With an ascent in osmolality, antidiuretic chemical delivery, this way, thirst is stimulated, so the organs retain water by lessening urinary discharge of water to the body, and drinking of water follows to reestablish plasma osmolality.

Of these two controlling structures, thirst is more significant. Indeed, even in the nonappearance of antidiuretic chemicals coming about a failure to reserve water, the thirst drive is adequate to permit support of an ordinary plasma sodium focus, yet to the detriment of the increasing polydipsia and polyuria. When a remarkably tolerant is denied admittance to water or cannot acquire water in light of some conditions, does the serum sodium focus rise, bringing about **hypernatremia**.

In the present circumstance of water deficiency, the sum of sodium in the extracellular liquid is significant; however, its fixation is expanded. The weakening of body solute by water, likewise with extreme water or excessively incredible organization of intravenous fluids, prompts hindrance of antidiuretic chemical delivery and water diuresis, again reestablishing plasma osmolality to ordinary.

Notwithstanding the osmolality control of vasopressin discharge, a sizable withdrawal of the extracellular liquid volume in the scope of 8 to 10% may likewise trigger the arrival of vasopressin and protection of water. A diminish in the potent blood volume, in any event, when the all-out extracellular liquid volume is expanded, may have a similar impact.

Suppose the standard components controlling the arrival of an antidiuretic chemical are disrupting under any circumstances. In that case, related infections, significant changes in the volume of the extracellular liquid, or organization of specific medications—water might be held. The weakening of the plasma solutes (i.e., hyponatremia) will result, regardless of whether the extracellular liquid's sodium substance is present.

With water shortfall, plasma sodium focus ascends; with water abundance, it falls, paying little mind to the extracellular liquid substance. Even though the plasma sodium fixation discloses nothing about extracellular fluid volume, it permits an induction with respect to intracellular volume. Expansion in plasma sodium (plasma osmolality) draws in the water out of the cell, prompting the intracellular volume's shrinkage. Hyponatremia (diminished plasma osmolality) permits the progression of water into the compartment and grows intracellular volume.

Since sodium is a significant osmotically dynamic molecule and since osmotic action changes oversee thirst and antidiuretic chemical delivery with resulting gain or loss of water, it could be seen that sodium content is vital in controlling the volume of the extracellular liquid.

An increase of sodium prompts chasing and holding water with the development of the extracellular liquid volume. At first, loss of sodium produces loss of water and withdrawal in the extracellular liquid volume. Consequently, sodium digestion oversees the volume of the extracellular liquid.

In well-being, the extracellular liquid volume development prompts renal sodium discharge; constriction of the extracellular liquid volume prompts renal protection of sodium. To be more exact, the withdrawal of the viable extracellular liquid volume or blood volume. The compelling blood volume is hard to characterize precisely; however, it appears to relate best to the blood vessel circuit's sufficient filling. This requires the upkeep of an acceptable cardiovascular yield, an adequate intravascular volume, and ordinary fringe opposition. A decreased cardiovascular yield hypoalbuminemia with a decrease in blood volume or an arteriovenous fistula all reduce the "totality" of the dissemination. Any of these conditions may prompt sodium maintenance. Such anomalies, when extraordinary, may flag sodium maintenance as well as antidiurctic chemical delivery that may prompt water maintenance and hyponatremia.

When this happens, the measure of sodium in the extracellular liquid is expanded, yet the fixation is decreased.

Accordingly, water digestion oversees the grouping of the extracellular liquid, although sodium digestion administers the volume of the extracellular fluid.

Hypernatremia

Hypernatremia results from an abundance of sodium. It is nearly consistent because of a shortage of water. In any case, high sodium abundance has happened in newborn children given unnecessary salt in their recipes. Once in a while, patients who have been given a lot of hypertonic sodium bicarbonate during some treatment or after cardiopulmonary capture may experience hypernatremia.

Formation of hypernatremia because of water deficiency is exemplified by the patient with debilitated or missing antidiuretic chemical delivery (focal diabetes insipidus) or kidney failure to react to antidiuretic chemical (nephrogenic diabetes insipidus). These two are somewhat exceptional circumstances and are not expected.

Most hypernatremia instances found in clinical practice are old patients with differing levels of debilitation of mental capacity. In this clinical setting, the pathogenesis of hypernatremia is not a failure to ration water; however, either a debilitated thirst drive or weakness with the powerlessness to acquire water. Such patients, except if malnourished, can think the urine typically, yet whenever handicapped or out of commission, is subject to some changes to give water. If the water level produced is deficient, particularly if expanded by fever or high natural temperatures, hypernatremia results. Some patients may have no view of thirst even with increments in plasma osmolality, yet this is an uncommon condition.

Indications of hypernatremia (and of hyponatremia) are of focal sensory system beginning and comprise of changes in points of view and the degree of cognizance. They identify with changes in the volume of the focal sensory system's cells (shrinkage with hypernatremia and growing with hyponatremia), significantly if the condition has proliferated. Water reduces, and hypernatremia deteriorates in hypernatremia patients, upset awareness prompting trance or disarray intensifies the issue because it is even more averse to look for or demand water. This arrangement may advance to irreversible neurologic harm and demise.

Treatment comprises of the organization of solute and water to reestablish plasma sodium and osmolality to ordinary.

Numerous patients with one or more hypo-or hypernatremia are asymptomatic. The two highlights that are of the best significance in deciding the presence or nonattendance of manifestations are the level of irregularity and the quickness with which the change has been created. Side effects in the fold from sodium fixation changes are surprising except if the sodium level is under 125 or over 160 mEq/L. Manifestations might be seen with lesser anomalies when they have been created in a couple of hours.

Hyponatremia

However, variation in plasma water may deliver clear, not real anomalies in plasma sodium, unreal hyponatremia. In hyperlipidemic states or with articulated hyperproteinemia, water content per unit volume of plasma is decreased. In these conditions, the plasma sodium fixation per liter of plasma water is ordinary. Still, since the decrease in water content, the sodium focus per liter of plasma is diminished.

Osmotic movement is ordinary, thirst and antidiuretic chemical delivery systems are undisturbed. The condition's significance lies in its acknowledgment so that it won't be mistaken for other hyponatremic states.

Hyponatremia may happen with the expansion of other osmotically dynamic particles, for example, glucose in uncontrolled diabetes mellitus or exogenous solutes like mannitol or glycerol, which are utilized as an osmotic diuretic or to bring down intraocular pressure in glaucoma, separately. In both these models, the presence of an osmotically active solute bound to the extracellular compartment draws in the water out of the system, weakening extracellular liquid and bringing down the sodium focus. Despite a diminished sodium level, osmolality is ordinary or expanded; this state could be named hypertonic hyponatremia.

In many occurrences, hyponatremia demonstrates hypotonicity: water abundance for the measure of sodium present. At the point when isotonic hyponatremia (hyperlipidemia or dysproteinemia) and hypertonic hyponatremia (hyperglycemia or exogenous solute) have been solved, it very well might be reasoned that lopsided water maintenance has happened and that hypotonic hyponatremia is the outcome.

Investigation of the pathogenesis and hyponatremia executives in the present condition is best drawn closer by evaluating the extracellular liquid volume. Evaluation of the extracellular liquid and intravascular volume is a clinical, not a research facility, assurance, albeit certain lab information (blood urea nitrogen and corrosive uric level) might be of help.

The highlights are isolating patients with hyponatremia into various classes dependent on the extracellular liquid. Think about first those patients with an extended extracellular liquid volume. The main highlight note is the presence or nonappearance of edema or ascites or indications of congestive cardiovascular breakdown like a dash.

In patients with a congestive cardiovascular breakdown or cirrhosis and ascites, hyponatremia is a generally late turn of events, so there is usually a background marked by prior edema or dyspnea to help the health practitioners in case of treatment. In these states, the edema liquid has a similar sodium focus as the plasma; the absolute body sodium is expanded. Lopsided maintenance of water, nonetheless, has prompted the weakening of the extracellular liquid solute.

Hyponatremia component in patients has been a subject of the discussion previously. Apparently, on many occasions, the arrival of antidiuretic chemicals because of a decrease in the intravascular volume is a significant contributor to water maintenance. Clinicians have discovered that these patients discharge water stacks inadequately and that imbuement of solute water, 5% dextrose in water, or hypotonic saline, may deliver or disturb hyponatremia. The components rely upon progress in the primary infection or limitation of water consumption. This methodology is fitting if hyponatremia is severe (under 120 mEq/L) or is indicative (modified degree of awareness).

When sodium is lost from the extracellular liquid, there is at first loss of water, and extracellular liquid volume is diminished. Loss of water happens in light of the fact that sodium reduces plasma osmolality and accordingly represses vasopressin discharge. The decreased osmolality of the extracellular liquid prompts water movement into the intracellular space. With moderate sodium changes, water is lost proportionately, and the plasma sodium level stays typical. If the sodium changes proceed and surpass around 200 mEq, the decrease in the extracellular liquid and plasma volume become adequate to trigger the arrival of antidiuretic chemical.

If the patient takes beverages or is given hypotonic fluid, water will not be discharged. This is forfeited for volume, water is held, and hyponatremia results.

In this condition, proper administration is transparent: substitution of sodium and water mixture. Supplanting is typically given with isotonic sodium arrangements; ordinary saline or one-half ordinary saline to which 45 mEq of sodium bicarbonate has been added is regularly utilized. Suggestive hyponatremia is phenomenal in this setting, yet if present, treatment with hypertonic saline is justified.

If water is held without sodium deficiency and within sight of a normal flow, there is a slight extension of the extracellular liquid volume and weakening of solutes, so hyponatremia results. Such a state might be mirrored by giving vasopressin to a typical subject over a few days.

More significant for clinicians, this state might be delivered by supported, self-governing arrival of vasopressin without the ordinary physiologic improvements, hyperosmolarity, or hypovolemia. In this sense, vasopressin's appearance is improper; accordingly, the nonexclusive name applied to this issue: the condition of unseemly antidiuretic chemical delivery (SIADH).

Since the underlying portrayal of this element in 1957, various SIADH instances of broadly different causes have been perceived. Supported arrival of vasopressin prompts water maintenance with the goal that plasma sodium level is decreased. Extracellular liquid volume is extended, bringing about sodium discharge in the urine (i.e., the urine is hypertonic to plasma and remains so regardless of extra water ingestion and further hyponatremia). A wide assortment of reasons for this condition has been recognized.

In the event that hyponatremia is amended to ordinary or close to typical levels inside a couple of hours, especially when the hyponatremic state has been of a few days' length, a disorder is described by significant neurologic incapacity may result. Signs range from simple conditions and conduct changes to quadriplegia with failure to swallow or talk. The morphologic difference to note is the loss of myelin in specific territories of the focal sensory system, especially the brain, henceforth the name focal pontine myelinolysis.

The significance of the pace of amendment of hyponatremia in this condition is discussed. Since the rise of the plasma sodium focus by just 5 or 6 mEq/L in patients with suggestive hyponatremia usually switches the neurologic anomalies, the further fast rise of the sodium level is not essential and might be unsafe.

Some extra reasons for hyponatremia ought to be referenced. In patients with intense oliguric renal changes, imbuements of hypotonic arrangements (5% dextrose in water or hypotonic saline) will prompt hyponatremia except if those arrangements are being given to supplant known conditions. In the present circumstance, the directed water "is directionless," and plasma sodium's weakening is the outcome.

Maniacal patients once in a while drink a lot of water, upward of 8 to 10 L each day. They may give hyponatremia, seizures, and trance. The pathogenesis is not clear in a significant number of these patients, even though a decrease of water admission, as a rule, amends the hyponatremic state and switches the indications.

Treatment with thiazide diuretics impedes the capacity to discharge water. They ought not to be endorsed in urgent water consumers beacuase suggestive hyponatremia with trance-like states or seizures can result.

A comparative succession might be seen in older patients given thiazide diuretics or given hypotonic liquids in the postoperative period. Certain medications may likewise impede water discharge and lead to hyponatremia:

- Chlorpropamide
- Vincristine
- Cyclophosphamide
- Clofibrate
- Carbamazepine

At long last, the plasma sodium level is diminished by around 4 mEq/L during pregnancy. The system of this decrease is not clear.

Chapter 6

6.0 Serum Magnesium

Magnesium is among the significant elements in the body. Like potassium, it performs several changes that are significant at both cellular and systemic levels. For example, magnesium is found to co-exist with many enzymatic reactors, thus called the cofactor. For example, it is located in the formation of adenosine triphosphate, where it plays a crucial role. Aside from this cellular function, magnesium function is seen in tissue functions and bone composition formation. About 70% of the bone composition is made of magnesium. This is while a person with hypomagnesemia shows many significant conditions which are dangerous to the individual.

Based on existence in the body, about 70% of the element is present in a free state, and the remaining percent is found as a compound in factors like phosphate, complex formers, and citrates.

The regulation of the element must be kept constant so that excess or reduced functionality of the substance will not cause havoc to the body. For example, excess stimulation of some proteins may be directly due to the action of hypermagnesemia, which is not hygienic. Thus, regular magnesium occurs in the kidney, especially in the ascending loop of Henle.

Magnesium reference values according to age differences (in years)

Adult >17	1.7 - 2.3 mg/dL
12 - 17	1.6 - 2.3 mg/dL
9 - 11	1.6 - 2.4 mg/dL
6 - 8	1.6 - 2.5 mg/dL
3 - 5	1.6 - 2.6 mg/dL
0 - 2	1.6 - 2.7 mg/dL

Hypomagnesemia

Significant contributors to a high level of magnesium in the blood are impaired regulation and influence of chronic conditions like chronic renal failure and acute conditions. The effect of magnesium may lead to depression, respiratory arrest, and cardiac arrest. On average, the deficiency in magnesium results in changes in the level of potassium, calcium, and phosphate in the blood. Moreover, this significantly affects overall body balance in coronary artery spasms, increased sensitivity to digoxin, among others.

Magnesium is a co-factor in numerous biochemical responses. Magnesium directly affects different electrolytes, including sodium, calcium, and potassium. As depicted above, low degrees of magnesium can happen optional to renal and gastrointestinal misfortunes.

Magnesium homeostasis includes the kidney (primarily through the proximal tubule, the thick rising circle of Henle, and the distal tubule), little gut (principally through the jejunum and ileum), and bone Hypomagnesemia happens when something, whether a medication or an infection condition adjusts the homeostasis of magnesium.

Magnesium inadequacy additionally can cause hypocalcemia, as the two are bury related. Decreased magnesium causes impeded magnesium subordinate adenyl cyclase age of cyclic adenosine monophosphate (CAMP), diminishing the arrival of parathyroid chemical (PTH). In turn, calcium levels are decreased just as PTH directs calcium levels.

Magnesium also influences the electrical activity of the myocardium and vascular tone, which is why patients with hypomagnesemia are in danger of heart arrhythmias.

Several conditions are seen in a patient with hypomagnesemia, and the common ones are listed below:

Hormone and electrolyte abnormalities	Includes hypokalemia, hypoparathyroidism, and hypocalcemia.
Cardiovascular changes	Atrial fibrillation, cardiac ischemia, ventricular and atrial premature systoles, ECG changes like peaked T waves.
Neuromuscular changes	Vertical nystagmus, apathy, seizures, tremors, tetany, delirium, and coma.

The average amount of magnesium in the body is around 1.46 - 2.68 mg/dL. The condition occurs when there is a low amount of magnesium in the blood, on a total serum magnesium level. This condition—hypomagnesemia may cause some impaired reaction in the nerve conduction, cellular function, among others. Hypomagnesemia leaves symptoms like cardiac ischemia abs mild tremors in a patient. Typical hypomagnesemia contributes to gastrointestinal losses, renal losses, chronic disease, and alcohol use disorder.

Conditions that induced/promotes hypomagnesemia

Gastrointestinal/renal induction, which leads to hypomagnesemia, includes	Gastric bypass surgery, acute pancreatitis, acute diarrhea, chronic diarrhea, inherited tubular disorder, familial hypomagnesemia, hungry bone syndrome.
A secondary cause of hypomagnesemia	Alcohol use disorder, starvation, and patient with parenteral diets
A secondary cause of hypomagncsemia (medications)	Amphotericin B, loop diuretics, thiazide diuretics, digitalis, chemotherapeutic drugs, and proton pump inhibitors.

Differential Diagnosis of hypomagnesemia

A comparative analysis is employed in treating a low amount of magnesium in the blood. In this case, other electrolytes are compared to magnesium as a low amount of magnesium can equally cause a low amount of calcium and potassium, as the case may be.

Management of hypomagnesemia

The treatment of hypomagnesemia patients depends on a patient's kidney work, the seriousness of their manifestations, and hemodynamic solidness. If a patient is hemodynamically unsteady in an intense clinic setting, 1 to 2 grams of magnesium sulfate can be given in around 15 minutes. For indicative, extreme hypomagnesemia in a steady tolerant, 1 to 2 grams of magnesium sulfate can be allowed more than one hour. Non-new repletion of the grown-up quiet is by large 4 to 8 grams of magnesium sulfate given more than 12 to 24 hours gradually. In pediatric patients, the portion is 25 to 50 mg kg (with a limit of 2 grams).

An asymptomatic patient who is not attended to or hospitalized and can endure drugs by mouth supported oral delivery substitution should be attempted first.

After repletion, serum electrolyte levels should be reevaluated (regardless of whether inpatient or outpatient) to guarantee that the treatment was effective. Although serum magnesium levels rise rapidly with treatment, intracellular magnesium takes more time to loaded.

Thus, patients with typical renal capacity should attempt to proceed with magnesium repletion for two days after the level standardizes.

Use alertness in replanting magnesium in patients with unusual kidney work (characterized as creatinine level under 30 ml min 1 73 m2). These patients are in danger of hypermagnesemia.

Studies suggest decreasing the magnesium portion by half and intently observing magnesium levels in these patients.

The hidden reason for tenacious hypomagnesemia ought to be tended to and treated. For instance, if a patient is reliably having low electrolyte levels because of renal misfortunes, they may profit from amiloride, potassium, and magnesium saving diuretic.

Hypermagnesemia

Hypermagnesemia occurs as an electrolytic disorder in the blood. The term happens when the level of magnesium is high than average in the blood. Several cases occur after the condition and are widely characterized by decreased breathing rate, confusion, weakness, low blood pressure, or even cardiac arrest.

On average, an impaired kidney is commonly the cause of hypermagnesemia, and this happens when the kidney fails to filter off excess magnesium in the body. Other reasons may be due to seizure, tumor lysis syndrome, and prolonged ischemia. When the blood level is higher than 2.6 mg/dL, a typical hypermagnesemia is confirmed in the body.

Causes of hypermagnesemia vary in individuals, and it might include:

- **Magnesium toxicity** occurs during labor and delivery and is directly linked to emergency pre-eclampsia treatment.

- **Chronic kidney disease**, at this point, the level of creatinine clearance just have called below 30 ml/min, and excretion of magnesium would have been impaired. Not all chronic kidney disease is characterized by hypermagnesemia, and unless magnesium is widely administered, this cannot be used as a cause.

- **Hemolysis,** when hemolysis occurs, the red blood cells divide. On average, the amount of magnesium in the red blood cells is higher than plasma magnesium. When excess blood is divided, more magnesium is produced from the blood and absorbed as plasma magnesium. Unless high hemolysis occurs, it cannot be a cause.

Diminished renal discharge

Hypermagnesemia happens essentially in patients with an intense or ongoing kidney infection. In this case, a few conditions, including proton siphon inhibitors, malnourishment, and liquor abuse, can build the chance of hypermagnesemia.

Hypothyroidism and particularly cortico-adrenal inadequacy are other perceived causes.

Hyperparathyroidism and changes in calcium digestion, including hypercalcemia and additionally hypocalciuria, can prompt hypermagnesemia through expanded calcium-instigated magnesium retention in the tubule. Patients with familial hypocalciuric hypercalcemia (FHH), an uncommon autosomal predominant condition, can show hypermagnesemia.

Lithium-based psychotropic medications can likewise prompt hypermagnesemia by lessening discharge.

Expanded admission

The issue may seldom grow even without renal hindrance, generally in the older, where an essential internal condition may prompt expanded retention through diminished gut motility. Patients treated with anticholinergics or narcotics or those with fiery gut infections are at higher risk.

For example, a few medications, diuretics and acid neutralizers that contain magnesium (e.g., magnesium oxide), can prompt expanded estimations of magnesium, particularly in old patients with renal capacity hindrance. E. g., the case of bioavailability makes magnesium oxide generally protected; its drawn-out use may prompt dangers of hypermagnesemia. Periodic assessment is a proposal in geriatric patients treated with magnesium oxide for expanded periods. Ultimately, magnesium oxide consumption under 1000 mg/day is by all accounts generally safe.

Serious hypermagnesemia has additionally been depicted after the organization of gut readiness specialists (e.g., sodium picosulphate magnesium citrate). Moreover, excessive oral admission can prompt hypermagnesemia in patients on hemodialysis, as ingestion fundamentally impacts these patients' plasma levels.

Patients with milk-salt disorder because of the ingestion of many calcium and absorbable antacid are more powerless to hypermagnesemia.

Since magnesium helps the administration of eclampsia (e.g., remedial serum magnesium level 1.7 to 3.5 mmol/L), the exorbitant imbuement can incite iatrogenic hypermagnesemia. Infants who have gotten magnesium sulfate parenterally during work may give poisonousness even with ordinary serum magnesium levels.

Compartment move or break

Magnesium levels increases in hemolysis patients. Red platelets contain threefold the amount of magnesium when contrasted with plasma. The burst of these cells empties magnesium into the plasma. Nonetheless, indicative hypermagnesemia happens just on account of forceful hemolysis.

Tumor lysis disorder, rhabdomyolysis, and acidosis (e.g., decompensated diabetes with ketoacidosis) can likewise incite hypermagnesemia through extracellular movements.

Renal capacity assumes a critical part in the digestion of magnesium. Of note, just around 10% of sifted magnesium is invested in the proximal tubule. In contrast, most of the separated magnesium gets latently reabsorbed in the rising appendage of the loop of Henle.

This factor is fundamental for the pathophysiology of kidney-related hypermagnesemia as along the loop of Henle, not just the volume of the filtrate gets diminished. Additionally, the osmolarity decreases essentially (- 66%), and this way, the solutes become less thought. Besides, this clarifies the high resorbent limit of the kidney, which by and large keeps up magnesium harmony until the creatinine leeway falls under 20 ml/min. Hence, an expansion in plasma magnesium levels is difficult to accomplish with diet alone in states of exceptional renal wellbeing.

Notwithstanding, the chances of hypermagnesemia increases by taking portions of magnesium. The pathophysiology of hypermagnesemia identified with abundance diuretic use is extraordinary. For this situation, the tremendous measure of magnesium given through the stomach-related parcel can prompt be overpowering the excretory component, particularly in cases with hidden subclinical renal changes.

Magnesium functions as a physiologic calcium blocker, expanded levels decide generous electrophysiological and hemodynamic impacts. Besides, the possible concomitance of hyperkalemia builds the danger of heart arrhythmias and heart failure.
The neurologic signs are the aftereffect of the restraint of acetylcholine discharge from the neuromuscular endplate because of expanded extracellular magnesium levels.

Patients with indicative hypermagnesemia can introduce distinctive clinical appearances relying upon the level and the time wherein the electrolytic aggravation has happened. Hypermagnesemia is, by and large, very much endured.

- Consequently, patients with modified qualities (under 4 mg/dL) might be asymptomatic or paucisymptomatic. The most successive indications and signs may incorporate shortcomings, queasiness, and disarray (under 7.0 mg/dL).

- Expanding values (7 to 12 mg/dL) incite diminished reflexes, deteriorating confusional state, bladder loss of motion, flushing, cerebral pain, and blockage. A slight decrease in circulatory strain and obscured vision brought about by reduced convenience and union can show.

- For higher qualities (over 12.0 mg/dL), muscle loss of motion, disabled ileus, diminished breathing rate, low circulatory strain, electrocardiogram (ECG) changes remembering an increment for PR and QRS stretch with sinus bradycardia, and atrioventricular square, trance state and heart failure (surpassing 15.0 mg/dL) may happen.

- When related to hypocalcemia, hypermagnesemia may initiate and form developments and seizures. The clinical picture turns out to be especially serious, and there are not many case reports of patients who are made due to higher hypermagnesaemia levels.

Treatment/the executives

Patients with typical renal capacity (GFR more than 60 ml/min) and gentle asymptomatic hypermagnesemia require no treatment aside from the expulsion of all wellsprings of exogenous magnesium. One should consider that the half-season of disposal of magnesium is roughly 28 hours.

In more extreme cases, close observing of the ECG, pulse, and neuromuscular capacity and early treatment is essential:

- Intravenous calcium gluconate or chloride [Dosage: 1 g in 2 to 5 min (repeatable more than 5 minutes)]. The reasoning is that the activities of magnesium in neuromuscular and cardiovascular capacity become estranged by calcium.

- Intravenous typical saline (e.g., at 150 ml/hour)

Clinical severe conditions require expanding renal magnesium discharge through:

- Intravenous circle diuretics (e.g., furosemide 1 mg/kg), or

- Hemodialysis, when kidney work is weakened, or the patient is indicative of extreme hypermagnesemia. This methodology generally eliminates magnesium productively (up to half decrease following a 3-to 4-hour treatment). Dialysis can, nonetheless, increment the discharge of calcium by creating hypocalcemia along these lines, potentially demolishing the manifestations and indications of hypermagnesaemia.

- The utilization of diuretics should be related to implantations of saline answers to dodge further electrolyte aggravations (e.g., hypokalemia) and metabolic alkalosis.

The clinician should perform sequential estimations of calcium and magnesium. In relationship with electrolytic remedies, it is frequently vital to help cardiorespiratory action. As an outcome, this electrolyte issue's therapy can require emergency unit admission as often as possible.

Specific clinical conditions require a particular methodology. For example, during eclampsia administration, the magnesium mixture is halted if urine yield drops to under 80 mL (in 4 hours), deep ligament reflexes are missing, or the respiratory rate is under 12 breaths/minute. A 10% calcium gluconate or chloride arrangement (10 mL intravenously repeatable more than 5 minutes) can fill in as a cure.

Chapter 7

7.0 Serum Calcium

Calcium remains the most bountiful element in the human body. In the total weight of a human, calcium weighs about 98% of the 1200g of calcium in an adult, and this exists in the form of hydroxyapatite in the skeleton. The combination of hydroxide, calcium, and phosphorus makes up the constitution of hydroxyapatite. Aside from the skeletal calcium, calcium is found in the extracellular fluid (about 50%) and other parts of the body, especially those with tissues responsible for various processes related to skeletal muscle. In the body, calcium should be at the range of 8.5 - 10.5 mg/dl, and this is considered the normal range of calcium in the body.

A slight deviation from this results in an abnormality of the substance. Aside from laboratory changes in the testing of calcium which might be as (0.5 mg/dl), high accuracy of the values should be maintained.

To be exactly accurate with calcium and its function, the lowest value is considered the right one due to various things that might cause value differences. For example, some triggers can lead to a high amount of calcium in the blood, and such serum calcium is considered false values in reality. Besides, the need for multiple calcium tests is reinforced due to the high chances of getting false values as far as calcium is concerned. This kind of value is mostly seen in patients dealing with high liver or renal failure and hemolysis conditions.

Possible causes that increase calcium levels in the blood are:

- **Venous occlusion of the arm.** During venipuncture, the arm is punctured, and this may increase the level of total blood calcium, even up to 0.3 mmol/L. Changes in hemodynamics lead to plasma protein distortion and thus creating a high level of calcium in the body.

- **Standing position.** Patients that are in a standing position may experience an increase in the level of blood calcium due to erecting supine position. And the increase ranges from 0.05 - 0.20 mmol/L

- **Contribution via an error in hemolysis**. High level of hemoglobin might contribute to high concentration of calcium after prolonged contact in the body. In case the error is due to hemolysis, new blood should be taken after overnight fasting, and the patient should not take any diets that might increase calcium levels in the blood again.

Functionality of calcium

The capacity of protein in relation to calcium goes about as support that modifies the impact of an intense load of calcium on the centralization of ionized calcium by about half. Still, another outcome of the significant number of unfilled restricting locales for calcium is that opposition by magnesium does not significantly affect ionized calcium focus.

The most crucial boundary influencing protein restricting calcium is the pH. An alkalemic pH prompts an increment in restricting and a decline in the small portion of ionized calcium. The purpose behind this is twofold:

- Inequalities among H^+ and Ca^{++} for restricting locales

- Modification in the setup of the egg white particles.

The plasma level of complexed calcium is typically assessed by the contrast between ionized and ultra-filterable calcium. As implied above, complex calcium comprises ionic couplets with anions like HCO_3^+ and HPO_4^+ and natural particles like lactate and citrate.

The most bountiful structure by all indications is $CaHCO^+{}_3$. As a result, there is as yet another system whereby pH adjusts the ionized calcium focus. An ascent in pH prompts an expansion of HCO_3, which at that point frames more complexed $CaHCO^+{}_3$, and consequently a fall in ionized calcium.

A takeoff of 1.0 g/dl from the ordinary egg white fixation will represent an adjustment of the protein-bound calcium division and, subsequently, the all-out calcium level of about 0.8 mg/dl.

The homeostatic calcium framework relies upon a few significant components: parathyroid chemical (PTH), nutrient D, phosphate, and magnesium.

PTH fills in as a receptor arm to address changes in the consistent state level of serum calcium.

A little fall in ionized calcium will rapidly prompt an ascent in PTH emission. The consequence of this increment in PTH is a quick arrival of calcium from bone. This delivery requires the dynamic type of nutrient D, 1,25-dihydroxycholecalciferol (1,25-DHCC); however, it is not subject to bone changes or an expansion in the number of osteoclasts.

This impact of PTH most presumably is intervened by means of the vehicle of calcium from the bone extracellular liquid (ECF). Just if the prerequisite for calcium is adequate bone-dry delayed, does PTH influence osteoclast expansion and increment bone changes.

PTH additionally acts to keep up the consistent state level of serum calcium by its activity on the kidney. It expands the cylindrical reabsorption of calcium and magnesium and diminishes the rounded reabsorption of phosphate, sodium, bicarbonate, potassium, and amino acids. PTH initiates the adenylate cyclase framework by restricting with receptor locales in the renal cortex. It subsequently prompts an increment in cyclic *adenosine monophosphate*.

Nutrient D builds the centralization of serum calcium by a few components. As referenced above, it potentiates the impact of PTH on the bone. Nutrient D additionally builds the intestinal assimilation of calcium, just as bone resorption and the overall reabsorption of calcium. The consequences for intestinal reabsorption of calcium and bone resorption appear to be expected essentially to the dynamic metabolite 1,25-DHCC.

Yet, different metabolites may add to a portion of different impacts on serum calcium.

Likewise, the serum phosphorus level assumes a part in supporting a uniform state convergence of serum calcium. While there is no definite solvency item for calcium and phosphorus, an ascent in serum phosphate, as a rule, prompts a fall in serum calcium.

A portion of this decrement might be brought about by the upgraded arrangement of CaHPO4 edifices in the serum. A fall in the degree of serum phosphate will alternately prompt an increment in the serum ionized and bone ECF calcium. A portion of the instruments that add to the drop of calcium incorporate.

The significance of ordinary serum calcium fixation can best be valued by a survey of the clinical appearances of hypocalcemia and hypercalcemia. The previous regularly prompts tetany, convulsive seizures, and cardiovascular, mental, and an assortment of ectodermal impacts. Hypercalcemia is generally connected with delicate tissue calcification, tubulointerstitial nephropathy, anorexia, sickness, electrocardiographic unsettling influences, and a range of neurologic changes from migraine to unconsciousness.

Expanded neural edginess is a genuinely regular sign of hypocalcemia. For the most part, the patient portrays shivering of the tips of the fingers and around the mouth. If it is unabated, these manifestations progress in seriousness and reach out to the appendages and face. The patient may likewise depict deadness over these territories that might be joined by carpal fit.

The greater part of these patients will have a positive Chvostek's and additionally Trousseau's sign.

Hypocalcemia may build focal, just as fringe, neural edginess, and two sorts of convulsive seizures may result. In the first place, the patient may experience the ill effects of a seizure issue like a patient without hypocalcemia, for example, petit mal, jacksonian, or fantastic mal.

Second, fundamental tetany may advance to delayed tonic fits, which are additionally alluded to as cerebral tetany.

The most well-known cardiovascular signs of hypocalcemia include unsettling influences of the electrical cadence. A fall in serum calcium will transpose ventricular repolarization and, in the process, increment the Q-T span and ST section. This may advance and create a 2:1 heart block. Persistent hypocalcemia may likewise prompt not exactly sufficient heart execution related to a decrease in pulse.

An assortment of mental appearances may go with hypocalcemia: these incorporate psychoneurosis, psychosis, and a natural mind disorder. Following the parathyroid medical procedure and the advancement of hypocalcemia and hypomagnesemia, an intense psychosis may create described by mental trips and distrustfulness. These are reversible on the remedy of the electrolyte aggravations.

A few imperfections of the ectoderm are regularly found in patients with ongoing hypocalcemia. Builds of water are the most widely recognized element.

This outcome from a change of the nearby sodium pump with possible focal point degeneration and the improvement of dystrophic calcifications. Deformities of the polish of teeth may happen if the hypocalcemia goes before the development of the separate tooth. Hair and nails may likewise be influenced by constant hypocalcemia. Both may get dry and fragile; their development may even be hindered.

Even more unordinary impacts of hypocalcemia may happen. These include aggravations of blood coagulation, intestinal malabsorption, inadequate bone mineralization (when related to nutrient D lack), optional hyperparathyroidism in the early stage of a hypocalcemic mother, slight papilledema, and calcification of the basal ganglion.

The indications, and thus the clinical importance, of hypercalcemia comprise of five impacts:

- delicate tissue calcification
- tubulointerstitial renal illness
- anorexia and queasiness
- Q-T prolongation of the electrocardiogram
- intense mind condition

Three locales of delicate tissue calcification happen with hypercalcemia even without serum phosphate increase. These are corneal and additionally conjunctival calcification, chondrocalcinosis, and renal calcification. While corneal calcifications are generally asymptomatic, conjunctival calcifications frequently are very bothering.

Keratopathy is a particular element brought about by dystrophic calcification regularly in hypercalcemia, however more uncommon than both of different types of calcification. Calcium pyrophosphate joint inflammation (i.e., chondrocalcinosis) has an expanded occurrence in the hypercalcemia of hyperparathyroidism (HPTH), yet not in different types of hypercalcemia.

The clinical qualities of hypercalcemic renal sickness incorporate a mild to direct fall in creatinine level, mild to direct rise of pulse, mild proteinuria, and hindered thinking capacity related to polyuria and nocturia. Pathologic changes ordinarily comprise interstitial fibrosis and medullary calcifications, which, if severe, show up as calcinosis by x-beam. An assortment of rounded dysfunctions may once in a while happen, notwithstanding those referenced. These incorporate glycosuria, phosphaturia, weakened potassium reabsorption, and improved hydrogen particle emission.

The most widely recognized gastrointestinal impacts of hypercalcemia incorporate anorexia, queasiness, and obstruction. The clogging is likely the consequence of parchedness and diminished hunger, while the queasiness is by all accounts a focal impact. The rate of ulcer sickness in HPTH stays disputable, while the recurrence of intense pancreatitis is by all accounts expanded in patients with HPTH.

Even though consistent state levels of serum calcium are imperative to myocardial capacity, cardiovascular anomalies related to hypercalcemia are restricted to shortening of the Q-T stretch, uncommon scenes of heart block, and an inclination to arrhythmias within sight of digitalis treatment. Hypertension is a genuinely basic impact of hypercalcemia and might be brought about by expanded fringe opposition as well as cardiovascular inotropism.

An intense mind disorder might be the most well-known symptom of moderate to extreme hypercalcemia. Side effects like sadness, persistent intermittent migraine, and memory impedance are regularly connected with ongoing hypercalcemia of mild to direct conditions. More articulated rises of serum calcium ordinarily lead to a range of side effects going from a mental disorder to a daze and trance state. The EEC regularly shows diffuse easing back reliable with metabolic encephalopathy.

Chapter 8

8.0 Serum Chloride

Chloride exists in the body; although it is an anionic element, it is imperative in the body, contributing to extracellular and intracellular changes. Notably, it is exclusively found in the extracellular fluid compartments, mixed with blood/plasma and the other interstitial fluids. In collaboration with sodium, chloride remains the major anion that collaborates with this substance. And its range from 96 - 106 mEq/L. On a significant trend, chloride is confined to the extracellular fluid, although some changes may lead it out of the cell, as the case may be.

The kidneys are answerable for the support of all-out body chloride balance. They keep up homeostasis because every kidney is made out of 1 million functional units, nephrons. Part of the chloride's entirety separated by the underlying bit of every nephron, the glomerulus, will be reabsorbed because of both dynamic and inactive motion measures along the tubules containing every nephron. The nephrons' capacity to reabsorb chloride keeps up the serum (and ECF) chloride focus inside a restricted reach.

Most of the separated chloride is reabsorbed with sodium during transportation through the tubule's main passage – the proximal tubule. The reabsorption of chloride in this portion happens in two stages.

In the underlying part of the proximal tubule, sodium passage into the cell is connected to dynamic co-transport of natural solutes (Na–glucose; Na–amino acids; Na–phosphate; and Na–natural anions) and to the active discharge of H+ from the tubule cells (and in this way the reabsorption of HCO3). Both of these dynamic cycles raise the intraluminal chloride fixation, creating, in the later fragments of the proximal tubule, the detached development of chloride and a good focus and electrochemical inclination. In the proximal tubule's straight pore, the standards recta, chloride reabsorption proceeds because of aloof dissemination down a great electrochemical level.

The end appendage of Henle's loop, the following pores of the nephron, is moderately impermeable to NaCl, and no Na or Cl drive happens. In the following portion, the thick rising appendage (circle of Henle), chloride is effectively moved by a particular transporter interceded cycle, and Na+ (or K+) follows latently to look after electro-neutrality.

The latest information recommends a model where two Cl– particles are moved for each Na+ and K+. Proof likewise proposes that chloride transport is additionally expanded in this section through the age of cyclic adenosine monophosphate by an antidiuretic chemical.

In the distal convoluted tubule, as in the proximal tubule, chloride transport might be latent or dynamic. It has been hypothesized, however not demonstrated, that chloride transport is coupled to the energy given by the aloof flood of sodium into the cell.

Other information recommends that the deliberate trans-epithelial potential contrast is adequately negative to clarify chloride development down a positive electrochemical inclination.

The last fragment of the nephron, the gathering conduit, is made out of three sections: the convoluted cortical tubule, the medullary convoluted tubule, and the convoluted papillary tubule. Chloride transport happens because of dynamic and detached cycles in the convoluted cortical tubules, yet by just dynamic drives measures in the papillary channel. No information is as of now accessible for the medullary conduit.

In summary, both dynamic and latent drive measures are significant in chloride reabsorption by the kidney's nephrons. The proximal tubule seems answerable for reabsorbing most of the separated chloride, and the climbing loop of Henle reabsorbs another critical sum. The distal tubule, in spite of the fact that reabsorbing a more modest amount of chloride, may likewise assume a significant part in this equilibrium.

Hyperchloremia

Hyperchloremia is additionally connected with an assortment of clinical conditions. Conditions causing a height of the serum chloride fixation and rise of the serum sodium focus result from messes related to loss of without electrolyte liquids (unmeasured water loss); hypotonic liquids (water shortfall in an overabundance of sodium and chloride deficiencies); or organization of NaCl-containing liquids.

Loss of electrolyte liquids happens in conditions with expanded apathetic loss because of expanded perspiring (e.g., fever); hypermetabolic states (thyrotoxicosis); raised surrounding room temperature and lacking water substitution (because of loss of thirst insight as found in the older); in sick babies; and in people with changed mental status (stroke patients, postanesthesia, and opiate drugs).

These outcomes in hypotonic drying out (e.g., loss of TBW and constriction of the ICF and ECF compartments) and a rise in both the serum sodium and chloride focus—hypernatremia and hyperchloremia. Loss of electrolyte liquids likewise happens in clinical conditions related to focal or nephrogenic diabetes insipidus.

The two conditions are associated with a failure to concentrate the urine and enormous diluted fluids (urine osmolality not as much as plasma osmolality).

Nonetheless, hypernatremia and hyperchloremia will not create in relationship with both of these last anomalies as long as people drink sufficient liquid measures or are given satisfactory amounts of intravenous electrolyte liquids to supplant everyday urine loss. Loss of hypotonic liquids happens with particular sorts of loose bowels states and consumes; in conditions related with an osmotic diuresis (e.g., diabetic glycosuria, mannitol, glycerol); diuretics; following a postobstructive diuresis, and in relation to certain characteristic renal infections.

Since more water is lost compared with sodium, the serum sodium chloride fixation rises. However, since some sodium and chloride are discharged into the urine, the serum sodium and chloride fixations will not be just about as raised as that happening in conditions related to loss without electrolyte liquids.

The organization of NaCl-containing liquids can likewise bring about hypernatremia and hyperchloremia if excessive amounts of hypertonic arrangements of sodium chloride (3 or 5%) are given iatrogenically instead of 5% D5/W or unintentionally directed during instillation in utero briefly semester fetus removal. It can likewise be found in a relationship with saltwater suffocating.

Organization of hypertonic cylinder feedings without the simultaneous organization of sufficient amounts of free water to weaken the feedings to isotonicity can likewise cause hypernatremia and hyperchloremia.

People with hyperchloremia auxiliary to electrolyte liquid loss will have actual discoveries of lack of hydration: dry mucous layers, covered tongue, and no axillary perspiration. Urine chloride and sodium focuses might be useful. Nevertheless, the finding of a weakened pee (Uosm under 100 mOsm with low chloride and sodium fixations) within sight of hyperchloremia and hypernatremia no doubt affirms the analysis of diabetes insipidus.

With the deficiency of hypotonic liquids, patients will face both a lack of hydration (a consequence of electrolyte liquid misfortunes) and sodium consumption.
As a result of the last mentioned, such people will have proof of ECF withdrawal (hypotension, tachycardia, orthostatic hypotension) furthermore. Interestingly, people with hyperchloremia optional to the NaCl-containing arrangements will have actual characteristics of an extended ECF volume: hypertension, edema, congestive cardiovascular breakdown, and pneumonic edema.

Raised degrees of serum chloride without expanded degrees of serum sodium happen because of clinical conditions that incline to hyperchloremic metabolic acidosis. People with this corrosive base aggravation have a serum chloride focus over 110 mEq/L (and a low bicarbonate fixation) in relationship with acidemic blood (pH lower than 7.35).

Hyperchloremic metabolic acidosis can happen when the kidney tubules (either proximal or distal) do not reabsorb sufficient amounts of the bicarbonate sifted by the glomerulus. Issues doing natural harm in the tubules (e.g., interstitial nephritis); tranquilizes that block bicarbonate reabsorption (e.g., carbonic anhydrase inhibitors—acetazolamide; and topically applied sulfur drugs and their metabolites utilized as a skin anti-infection in consume patients) bring about the condition called rounded renal acidosis (RTA).

A conclusion of RTA can now and again be made if one finds a blood pH that is acidemic in relationship with nonacidic urine (a urine pH above 5.5).

Different reasons for hyperchloremic metabolic acidosis incorporate conditions related with extreme the runs having misfortunes of bicarbonate counterparts (e.g., lactate and acetic acid derivation); ureteral redirection systems, which frequently have hyperreabsorption of chloride by the mediated inside section; and ingestion of acidic chloride-containing salts (NH_4Cl, arginine chloride, and lysine chloride); or acidic salts of amino acids found in some hyperalimentation arrangements. Hyperchloremic metabolic acidosis can likewise be found in the beginning phases of constant renal disappointment, particularly auxiliary to conditions coming about because of interstitial renal harm; in the healing period of diabetic ketoacidosis (deficiency of ketone bodies in the urine keeps them from being changed over to bicarbonate in the liver and results in bicarbonate shortages); and in essential hyperparathyroidism (which is related with renal bicarbonate misfortunes). Similarly, respiratory alkalosis, a condition found in people with hyperventilation (e.g., sepsis, pregnancy, pneumonic diseases, nervousness), is related to a raised serum chloride focus and a low bicarbonate fixation. A blood vessel's blood pH will help recognize hyperchloremic metabolic acidosis and respiratory alkalosis.

Hyperchloremia is additionally seen with bromide inebriation since bromide is estimated as a chloride comparable by specific chloride estimation strategies. These outcomes in the finding of an anion hole (as evaluated by the distinction of sodium and potassium short chloride in addition to the absolute CO_2 content being under 8 mEq/L).

Albeit the utilization with bromide has diminished, instances of bromide inebriations happen. It is surprising to see intense bromide inebriation since bromide causes critical gastrointestinal aggravation, bringing about sickness and regurgitating, making harmful levels hard to accomplish.

Moderate constant ingestion of bromide, be that as it may, can prompt toxic levels since the kidneys discharge bromide, and equilibrium can happen if allowed to surpass yield. The clinical highlights of bromide inebriation incorporate fever, neurologic aggravations, skin rash, and a history of ingesting restrictive bromide-containing drugs.

The toxic appearances include sedation, unsettling clairvoyant influences, quakes, system incoordination, and expansions in CSF crucial factor and protein. Falsely expanded degrees of serum chloride fixation show up in bromism, yet the rising level is reliant on chloride utilization. There might be a helpless connection between the seriousness of bromide inebriation and serum bromide levels. Notwithstanding, bromide inebriation will cause mental and neurologic side effects when bromide serum levels surpass 9 mEq/L. Most patients indicate bromide effect when the serum bromide focuses are in the scope of 19 to 25 mEq/L.

Hypochloremia

Renal and external causes may lead to total body chloride loss. Some of the external causes include the inadequacy of sodium chloride intake to the body. When chlorine is not much in the body, the body cannot use the necessary amount to perform the regular function. Also, a shortage of chlorine due to external causes include loss of HCl in the body or diarrhea effects in the case of small bowel transport. When fluids are lost through the skin, it might lead to the loss of chlorine simultaneously. Vomiting may lead to must loss of chlorine compare to any other element.

This is because the gastric chloride content is higher than most gastric sodium elements, which directly influences the level or amount of chlorine that will be lost from a single pour of vomits in a patient. A patient with severe nasogastric may only show an average loss of sodium via vomiting, but the same contributes to a high average loss (80 to 90 mEq/L). Pernicious vomiting that is directly due to gastric outlet obstruction contributes to increased loss of serum chloride, and that is about (45 - 70 mEq/L). Self-induced vomiting contributes to high serum chloride loss, irrespective of the condition that leads to such vomiting action.

High loss of serum chloride shows in the physical sense of the patient. For example, condition like tachycardia, hypotension, and changes in blood pressure) maybe observed in a patient with hypochloremia—especially those that have rapid chloride depletion, as discussed so far. On average, the external loss of serum chloride is higher in volume compared to the renal loss. Notwithstanding, the importance of renal serum chloride loss should not be underrated.

Renal serum chloride loss is primarily contributed by osmotic diuresis, diuretic abuse, and loop diuretics. Many medical conditions are mainly associated with loss of serum chloride due to renal losses. The typical case of these conditions is that they all contribute to salt-losing nephropathy, which is: chronic renal failure, adrenal insufficiency, and post obstructive diuresis. The same determinants and signaling loss of chlorine will be noticed in individuals with external chlorine loss and renal failure. However, chloride urine concentration will be high in those with renal loss compared to individuals with external loss contributors.

Another finding regularly connected with chloride consumption is metabolic alkalosis (blood pH more prominent than 7.45). The reabsorption of sodium bicarbonate (NaHCO3) in the proximal and distal tubule is expanded. All out body chloride exhaustion brings about ECF volume compression (which animates HCO3 reabsorption) and diminished amounts of sifted chloride accessible to the tubules for reabsorption with sodium. The virtual shortfall of chloride in the urine within sight of metabolic alkalosis is a solid sign that total body chloride consumption is available.

Enlarged reabsorption of NaHCO3 will endure until sufficient amounts of chloride are managed, and the volume of the ECF compartment is standardized. Metabolic alkalosis additionally builds potassium discharge by the kidneys, which can prompt hypokalemia.

Various chloride-containing arrangements can be utilized to address all-out body chloride consumption, including isotonic sodium chloride (ordinary saline, physiologic saline) for substitution of just sodium and chloride; potassium chloride for substitution of potassium and chloride; and lysine monochloride, arginine monochloride, ammonium chloride, or HCl when corrosive substitution is vital in conditions related with chloride exhaustion and extreme metabolic alkalosis.

Clinical conditions related to abundance water maintenance can cause dilutional hyponatremia with a proportionate decline in the chloride level. This type of hypochloremia does not reflect complete body chloride or sodium exhaustion. Large numbers of the conditions related to dilutional hypochloremia have a typical or expanded all-out body substance of chloride and sodium.

For the most part, people with dilutional hypochloremia have an ordinary or raised circulatory strain and proof of ECF volume extension. The sodium and chloride urine focuses are variable, relying upon the primary ailment.

Explicit corrosive base anomalies may likewise be related to hypochloremia. Conditions associated with respiratory acidosis (e.g., maintenance of CO2 similarly as with persistent obstructive lung sickness) cause the proximal tubule to build its discharge of hydrogen particles. This outcome in sodium being held preferentially as sodium bicarbonate and not sodium chloride. Albeit this is a compensatory system to help enhance the acidemia, the outcome is expanded centralizations of serum bicarbonate (more prominent than 30 mEq/L) and diminished serum chloride fixations.

Conditions causing dilutional hyponatremia and hypochloremia do not need chloride-containing liquids since they do not have absolute body chloride consumption. Notwithstanding, respiratory acidosis related to hypochloremia may require chloride-containing fluids if metabolic alkalosis and hypokalemia are present.

Chapter 9

9.0 Arterial Blood Gases

The case of acid-base imbalance can often cause a high case of a severe condition in a patient. This can elongate to life-threatening issues and therefore the study of arterial blood gases is crucial to study. The act of knowing the arterial blood gases (ABG) is vital means of managing and diagnosing acid-base balance and the oxygenation status of the high-risk patients, also in patients that are admitted in intensive care Units of a hospital. Since the means of knowing and manipulating the arterial blood gases demands and requires a thorough understanding, it is therefore required a course for physicians and other medical practitioners. A wrong understanding as well as interpretation of acid-base balance mean a high life-threatening situation; this might directly demand patient life. Throughout this course, the need to study acid-base balance must be handled with a serious mind and soul. In order to finally understand the concept of acid-base balance, both study and impaction are required.

However, all this concept may not be included in single literature, especially the concept of Stewart's strong ion difference. Notwithstanding, this book covers significant measures in the image of acid-base balance.

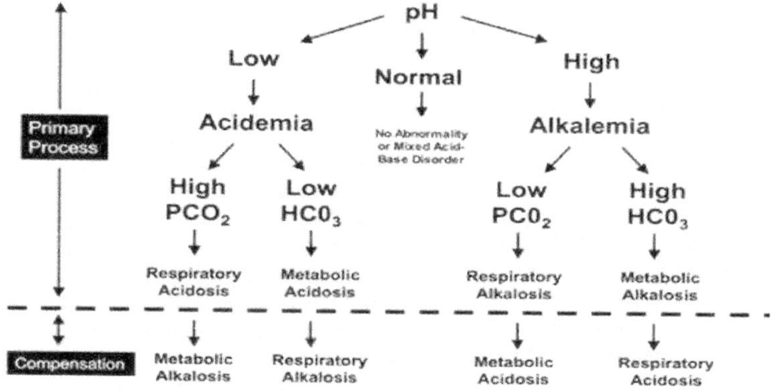

Introduction

Arterial blood gas (ABG) is a means of knowing and diagnosing the essential parts of the patient's oxygenation status, alongside the acid-base balance. The diagnosis is not as important as the ability to interpret the results of the ABG concept. In the processes involved in establishing a true ABG, interpreting the concept is the most crucial among all.

The three broadly utilized ways to deal with corrosive base physiology are the HCO3 (with regards to pCO2). Standard base excess (SBE) and vital ion difference (SID).

It has been a long time since Stewart's idea of SID was presented, characterized as the outright contrast between totally separated anions and cations. According to the guideline of electrical neutrality, this distinction is adjusted by weak acids and CO2.

The SID is characterized regarding weak acids and CO2 has been consequently re-assigned as compelling (SID), which is indistinguishable from "cradle base". Similarly, Stewart's unique term for complete feeble corrosive fixation (A_{TOT}) is currently characterized as the separated (A) or more undissociated (AH) frail acid structures. This is naturally known as anion gap (AG) when the ordinary focus is brought about by A^-.

Therefore, every one of the three strategies yields practically indistinguishable outcomes when utilized to evaluate the acid-base status of a given blood test.

Needs for ABG Analysis

The breakdown of ABG Analysis allows the medical practitioners to aid:

- Ventilator management
- Adjustments in acid/base balance and management
- The best treatment schedule
- In determining the correct diagnosis
- The acid/base status, which may alter electrolyte levels in critical conditions.

Perfect results for an ABG rely upon the appropriate way of extraction, handling as well as examining the sample.

Clinically significant blunders may happen at any of the above advances, yet ABG estimations are incredibly subjective to pre-analytic mistakes.

The most widely recognized issues that are experienced incorporate non-arterial tests, air rises in the sample, lacking or over the top anticoagulant in the sample, and deferred examination of a non-cooled sample.

Likely Pre-analytical Errors during ABG.

Pre-analytical errors are caused at the accompanying stages during ABG. For example:

- During arrangement preceding inspecting
- Absent or wrong quiet/example ID;
- Utilization of the off base sort or measure of anticoagulant
    - weakening because of the utilization of fluid heparin;
    - inadequate measure of heparin;
    - restricting of electrolytes to heparin;
- Lacking adjustment of the respiratory state of the patient; and
- Lacking evacuation of flush arrangement in blood vessel lines preceding blood assortment.

During testing/dealing with

- Combination of venous and blood vessel blood during penetrating

- Presence of air bubbles in the sample. Any air bubble in the sample should be removed straight away in the wake of pulling out the sample and before blending in with heparin or prior to any form of cooling the sample as the case might be.

  An air bubble whose overall volume is up to 1% of the blood in the needle is an expected means of critical mistake and may significantly influence the pO2 esteem.

- Inadequate blending in with heparin.

During stockpiling/transport

- Mistaken capacity
- Hemolysis of platelets

General Storage Recommendation

- Try not to cool the sample.
- Dissect inside 30 min. For tests with high paO2, e.g., shunt or with high leukocyte or platelet check additionally examine inside 5 min.
- When the examination is required to be postponed for over 30 minutes, utilization of glass needles and ice slurry is suggested.

During readiness preceding sample transfer

- Outwardly examine the example for clumps.
- Lacking blending of tests before the examination.

Lacking blending might cause coagulation of the example. It is prescribed to blend the blood test entirely by reversing the needle multiple times and moving it between the palms.

During anticoagulation

Current blood gas needles and fine cylinders are covered with different sorts of heparin to forestall coagulation in the sampler and inside the blood gas analyzer:

- Fluid non-balanced heparin
- Dry non-balanced heparin
- Dry electrolyte-adjusted heparin (Na+, K+, Ca2+)
- Dry Ca2+-adjusted heparin

Different anticoagulants, e.g., citrate and EDTA, are both marginally acidic, which increment the danger of pH being erroneously brought down

Interpretation of ABG results

In order to obtain relevant results from a patient, even after the test, the patient medical history must be examined. The history can commit the previous level of the situation, especially the given acid-base disorder's etiology. For example, metabolic acidosis may arise from ABG treatment if the patient has a history of hypotension, unmeasured diabetic status, or renal failure. Therefore, the medical record does not only contributes to the basis of getting the proper treatment for an ABG patient, but it also helps to prevent a condition that might arise as an aftermath of medical treatments. Likewise, metabolic alkalosis may be a direct issue to a patient with a medical history that includes high-nasogastric aspirate, vomiting, or bicarbonate administration.

During the test, the oxygen level of the patient needs to be observed. Regularly, the level of paO_2 is the direct determinant of oxygen levels. However, in this case, the level of FiO_2 must be calculated–this allows a smooth collaboration between the process. And the paO_2 level is used to classify the oxygen level as mild, moderate, or severe hypoxia.

Acid-base status

Acid-base status Identify the essential issue of ABG by taking a gander at the pH

pH > 7.40 = Alkalemia: 7.40 = Acidemia

At that point, take a gander at paCO2, which is a respiratory acid, regardless of whether it is expanded, i.e., >40 (acidosis) or diminished <40 (alkalosis), and assuming this clarifies the difference in pH, it is respiratory disorder; in any case, see the pattern of the progress of HCO_3^- (whether expanded in alkalosis or diminished in acidosis)– In the event that it clarifies the difference in pH, it is a metabolic problem.

In an ordinary ABG

- pH and paCO2 move in inverse ways.
- HCO3-and paCO2 move the same way.

- When the pH and paCO2 alter in a similar course (which typically ought not), the essential issue is metabolic; when pH and paCO2 move in inverse ways and paCO2 is normal, it is vital is respiratory.

- Mixed Disorder–if HCO3-and paCO2 alter in the inverse course (which they typically should not), at that point, it is a mixed problem: pH might be ordinary with strange paCO2 or unusual pH and typical paCO2).[7]

In the event that the pattern of progress in paCO2 and HCO3-is something similar, check the percent distinction. The one that has a more noteworthy % distinction between the two is the one that is the predominant issue.

e.g.: pH = 7.25 HCO3-=16 paCO2=60

Here, the pH is acidotic, and both paCO2 and HCO3- clarify its acidosis: so take a gander at the % distinction

HCO3-% distinction = (24 - 16)/24 = 0.33

paCO2% distinction = (60 - 40)/40 = 0.5

Chapter 10

10.0 Causes of Acid-Base Disturbances

Disorder	pH	HCO_3^-	Pco_2	Calculation for Compensation
Normal	7.40	24	40	
Metabolic acidosis	Decreased	Decreased	Decreased	Expected $Pco_2 = 1.5$ (serum HCO_3) + 8 ± 2
Metabolic alkalosis	Increased	Increased	Increased	$\Delta Pco_2 = 0.7 \times \Delta HCO_3$ or $Pco_2 = HCO_3 + 15$
Respiratory acidosis	Decreased	Increased	Increased	Acute: $\Delta HCO_3 = 0.1 \times \Delta Pco_2$ Chronic: $\Delta HCO_3 = 0.3 \times \Delta Pco_2$
Respiratory alkalosis	Increased	Decreased	Decreased	Acute: $\Delta HCO_3 = 0.2 \times \Delta Pco_2$ Chronic: $\Delta HCO_3 = 0.4 \times \Delta Pco_2$

Metabolic acidosis

Metabolic acidosis occurs as a condition where there is more than enough acid in the body fluids. When this happens, the perfect operatives processes in an acidic medium would be working perfectly; however, essential functions may be affected.

The major contributor to metabolic acidosis is when the kidney could not excrete more acids as they are produced in the body. Some of the conditions that also contribute to metabolic acidosis include:

- Kidney disease
- Lactic acidosis
- Severe dehydration
- Hyperchloremic acidosis

Symptoms

Most of the causes are directly related to some underlying disease and it is more significant to know what could result in metabolic acidosis and therefore prevent it with time. The certain determinant of metabolic acidosis is the aspect of rapid breathing. And other symptoms include shock, tiredness as well as feeling confused.

Examination and tests

The significance of these tests and examination is the distinguishable feature to outline where the cause is due to a metabolic problem or directly related to a breathing problem. And some of the test include:

- Urine ketones
- Urine pH
- Blood ketones
- Arterial blood gas

Metabolic alkalosis

Metabolic alkalosis is a condition when the body shows the excess base and opposite of metabolic acidosis.

Alkalosis occurs when there is a deviation in the level of acid-base balance in the body.
The kidney is the suitable organ that maintains this balance; however, when the body changes in a way that that there is a decreased number of carbon dioxide (an acid), or increased bicarbonates (a base) and metabolic alkalosis occurs.

Some of the conditions that contributes to metabolic alkalosis include the following:

- Lung disease
- Liver disease
- Staying at a high altitude
- Fever
- Aspirin poisoning

Symptoms

Symptoms of alkalosis can incorporate any of the accompanying

- Disarray (can advance to trance or trance-like state)
- Muscle jerking
- Prolonged muscle spasms
- Hand quake
- Vomiting and nausea
- Numbness or shivering in the face, hands, or feet
- Lightheadedness

Tests and Tests

The medical services supplier will play out an actual test and get some information about your indications

Lab tests that might be ordered incorporate

Blood vessel blood gas investigation

- Electrolytes test, for example, essential metabolic board to affirm alkalosis and show whether it is either respiratory or metabolic alkalosis

Different tests might be expected to decide the reason for the alkalosis. These may incorporate:

- Chest x-beam
- Urine pH
- Urinalysis

Respiratory acidosis

Respiratory acidosis is a condition or situation that occurs when the lungs cannot remove all the Co_2 in the body. And this results in body fluids being more acidic, especially in the blood.

Causes of respiratory acidosis

Causes of respiratory acidosis include the following:

- Obstructive sleep apnea
- Scoliosis and other diseases that affect the chest
- Pulmonary fibrosis, and some other diseases of the lung tissue, primarily cause scarring and thickening of the lungs.
- Conditions that attack the nerves and muscles that signal the lungs to either inflate or deflate.

The kidney may easily adjust the condition since it occurs over a long period. And, significantly, the kidney allows smooth acid-base balance with time. And this is notable in chronic respiratory acidosis.

In acute respiratory acidosis, the body combines more carbon dioxide before the kidney could eventually remove the excess ones. Therefore, it is more severe compared to chronic respiratory acidosis. A chronic respiratory acidosis patient may show acute respiratory acidosis symptoms later on, as this is more severe and disrupts the body's acid-base balance.

Symptoms

- Disarray
- Nervousness
- Simple weakness
- Laziness
- Languor
- Shaking
- Warm and flushed skin
- Perspiring

Examination and Tests

The medical services supplier will play out an actual test and get some information about manifestations.

Tests that might be done include:

- Blood vessel blood gas, which estimates oxygen and carbon dioxide levels in the blood
- Essential metabolic board
- Chest x-beam
- CT output of the chest
- Pneumonic capacity test to gauge breathing and how well the lungs are working

Respiratory alkalosis

Respiratory alkalosis occurs when there is a low level of carbon dioxide in the blood due to breathing excessively.

Causes

- Pain
- Tumor
- Panic or anxiety
- Pregnancy
- Severe anemia
- Liver disease
- Over breathing

Symptoms

- Dizziness
- Lightheadedness
- Numbness of both hands and feet
- Breathlessness
- Confusion
- Chest inconvenience

Your medical care supplier will perform an actual test.

- Blood vessel blood gas, which estimates oxygen and carbon dioxide levels in the blood
- Basic metabolic board
- Chest x-beam
- Aspiratory work tests to quantify breathing and how good the lungs are working

www.ingramcontent.com/pod-product-compliance
Ingram Content Group UK Ltd.
Pitfield, Milton Keynes, MK11 3LW, UK
UKHW021909190726
13853UKWH00002B/593